THE DURABLE PHYSIQUE

Build a Body That Lasts

J Leme Thompson

Medical Disclaimer

The information in this book is intended for educational purposes only and does not constitute medical advice. The content reflects the author's research and personal experience and is not a substitute for professional medical guidance, diagnosis, or treatment.

Before beginning any new exercise program, nutrition plan, or making significant changes to your diet, consult a qualified healthcare provider — particularly if you have any pre-existing medical conditions, are taking medications, or have concerns about your health.

The author and publisher assume no responsibility for any injury, loss, or damage incurred as a result of the use or application of information contained in this book.

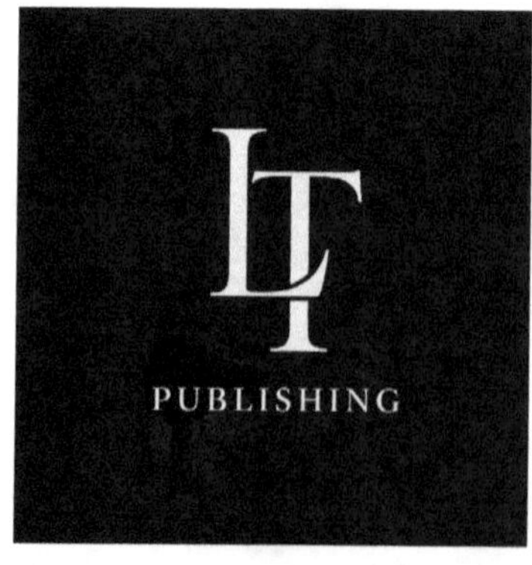

Crafted with patience and purpose

Dedication

For Alex, who taught me that eating more can be a good thing.

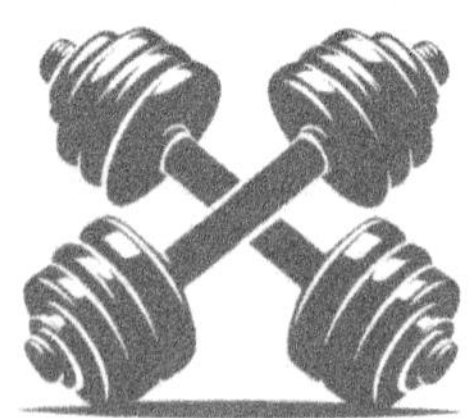

Note to Reader

This book was not written by a coach, a trainer, or a physiologist. It was written by someone who spent years running hard in the wrong direction.

For a long time, progress was treated as something to chase aggressively. Faster weight loss. Tighter rules. More urgency. Each new diet felt like a sprint—intense, exhausting, and briefly effective. Like the hare in the old fable, early speed created the illusion of winning. The scale moved quickly. Results felt real.

They never lasted.

What eventually became clear is that body composition does not reward speed. It rewards consistency, recovery, and patience. Muscle is slow to build and easy to lose. Fat loss that ignores this reality trades short-term success for long-term regression. The harder the sprint, the harder the rebound.

The alternative is quieter, but it is not easier. It requires discipline of a different kind. Not the discipline of constant restriction or emotional urgency, but the discipline to execute the same fundamentals—training, protein intake, carbohydrates, recovery—day after day without escalation when progress feels slow.

Tracking macros is a good example. It demands attention, honesty, and consistency. It is not optional if precision is required. But its purpose is not control for its own sake—it is alignment. Discipline here means hitting targets reliably, not tightening them reflexively. Staying steady instead of sprinting.

This approach resembles the tortoise—not because it lacks effort, but because it applies effort sustainably. Progress comes in small, often unimpressive increments. Strength is preserved. Habits stabilize. Results accumulate instead of resetting.

This book began as a way to understand why the sprint kept failing and what actually worked when the goal was permanence instead of speed. Over time, it became clear that the same pattern plays out for countless others: effort is high, discipline is real, but the strategy is mismatched to how the body adapts.

Everything that follows is built around a simple premise: progress that lasts must be disciplined, recoverable, and repeatable. There are faster ways to lose weight. There are harsher ways to suffer. This is about neither.

It is about applying discipline where it compounds—and having the restraint not to abandon it when progress feels quiet.

Introduction

If you lift weights consistently, eat reasonably well, and still look largely the same year after year, this book was written for you.

You are not lazy.

You are not undisciplined.And you are not broken.

What you are is stuck inside a system that was never designed for people like you.

Modern fitness culture offers two primary paths for changing your body:

1. **Bulk** — eat more, gain muscle, accept fat gain

2. **Cut** — eat less, lose fat, accept muscle loss

Repeat this cycle long enough and you're told progress is inevitable.

In real life, most natural lifters don't end up bigger, leaner, and stronger. They end up frustrated, smaller than they started, and perpetually dieting.

Some quit entirely.

This isn't because they failed the process.It's because the process failed them.

This book is written for:

- Natural lifters

- Adults with jobs, stress, families, and limited recovery

- People who train seriously but don't want their lives consumed by dieting

- Lifters who care about strength, performance, and appearance—not just scale weight

It is not written for:
- Competitive bodybuilders peaking for a stage

- Enhanced athletes with pharmaceutical recovery

- Influencers selling extremes

If your goal is to look leaner without shrinking, to maintain strength while losing fat, and to stop restarting every few months, you're in the right place.

An Inconvenient Truth

Most fat-loss advice treats muscle as collateral damage.

Lose weight fast. Worry about muscle later. "Just bulk again."

What this ignores is biological reality: muscle is expensive tissue. It requires energy to maintain, repair, and signal. When calories are aggressively restricted, the body prioritizes survival, not aesthetics. Muscle is not protected out of loyalty—it's protected only when conditions allow it.

In people who are already stressed, under-recovered, and training hard, those conditions don't exist. Cortisol stays elevated, recovery capacity shrinks, and the body looks for ways to reduce its energy burden. Lean mass becomes a logical target.

The loss is rarely dramatic. It's subtle and cumulative—a missed rep here, flatter muscles there, strength that's harder to regain each cycle. Over time, this quiet erosion reshapes the physique in the wrong direction.

Many lifters unknowingly diet themselves into worse body composition year after year: each cut is harsher, each rebound softer, and each "leaner" phase supported by less muscle than the one before. The scale may go down, but the frame underneath it keeps getting smaller:

They weigh less. They look flatter. They perform worse. Fat regain becomes easier.

This book exists to stop that cycle.

The Problem Recomposition Solves

Body recomposition is not magic. It doesn't rely on special genetics, secret protocols, or bending the rules of physiology. It is simply the result of applying known principles in the right context.

It is not beginner luck either. While beginners often experience it more easily, recomposition can occur at other stages when training is well-structured, recovery is sufficient, and nutrition supports both adaptation and fat loss. What changes with experience is the margin for error—not the mechanism.

And it does not violate energy balance. Fat loss still requires an overall energy deficit, and muscle growth still requires adequate energy and protein. Recomposition works by partitioning resources more effectively—using stored body fat to help cover the energy cost of building or preserving muscle while external intake is controlled.

When those conditions aren't met, recomposition stalls. When they are, it looks impressive—but it's still biology, not magic.

Recomposition is a strategy that prioritizes:

- Muscle retention first

- Fat loss second

- Sustainability always

Instead of asking, "How fast can I lose weight?"Recomposition asks, "How can I improve body composition without sacrificing strength or sanity?"

That shift changes everything.

The Reality of the Process

Recomposition is slower than crash dieting because it refuses to shortcut the process. It doesn't rely on extreme deficits, dehydration, or muscle loss to create rapid scale changes. Instead, it works within the body's actual limits—preserving lean mass while gradually reducing fat.

That restraint is exactly what makes it durable.

When recomposing, the scale often becomes a blunt tool. Expect weeks where it barely moves—not because nothing is happening, but because fat loss and muscle preservation (or even gain) are occurring simultaneously. Visual changes tend to show up first: a tighter waist, clearer muscle separation, clothes fitting differently. The numbers lag behind.

Strength maintenance becomes a key success metric. Holding performance under controlled intake is not stagnation—it's evidence that muscle is being protected. In many cases, simply not getting weaker is progress.

Most importantly, recomposition operates on a longer timeline. Progress is measured in months, not days. This demands patience, but it also produces outcomes that last: a better physique built on a stronger frame, not a lighter one.

If you're willing to trade speed for permanence, this approach works—quietly, predictably, and without the rebound that crash dieting almost always brings.

How to Use This Book

Read it in order.Do not skip ahead looking for shortcuts. Recomposition rewards patience and punishes panic.

Contents

Part I

Understanding Body Recomposition

Most people fail not because they lack discipline. They fail because they are following a system designed for someone else.

Bulk and cut cycles, scale obsession, and aggressive deficits are the default advice — and for most natural lifters, they reliably produce frustration, muscle loss, and diminishing returns.

This section explains why the standard approach fails, what body recomposition actually is, and how calories function in a system built for permanence rather than speed.

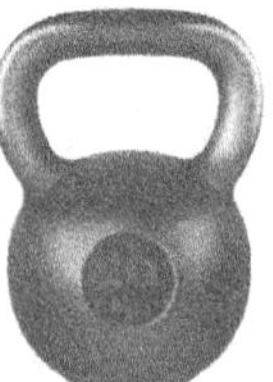

Chapter 1
Understanding Body Recomposition

Why Fat Loss Fails Most Lifters

Walk into any commercial gym and you'll see the same pattern repeated over and over. People show up week after week. They lift weights consistently, push through tough sessions, and leave drenched in sweat. Outside the gym, they try to eat "clean," avoid obvious junk, and follow the advice they've been told is responsible and effective.

And yet, months go by with little to show for it.

Some get weaker instead of stronger. Some look smaller rather than leaner. Many grow frustrated and eventually quit altogether.

This isn't a lack of effort or discipline. It's a framework problem. When the framework is wrong, consistency stops compounding and starts wearing people down instead. Most lifters are doing exactly what they were told would work—train hard, eat clean, stay consistent—only to discover that effort alone doesn't guarantee progress. When the underlying strategy is flawed, working harder simply accelerates burnout, not results.

Without a system that aligns training, nutrition, and recovery toward a clear goal, consistency becomes directionless. The problem isn't that people aren't trying hard enough. It's that they've been given a plan that doesn't work for how they live, train, and recover in real life.

The Bulk/Cut Trap Traditional fitness culture teaches that progress must occur in rigid phases: bulk to gain muscle and accept fat gain, then cut to lose fat and accept muscle loss. On paper, this appears logical. In practice, it fails most non-elite lifters.

Bulking often drifts into unchecked overeating. The surplus stops being intentional and starts being justified, while fat gain accelerates faster than any measurable increase in strength. Fat gain accelerates faster than muscle growth, creating a larger problem to solve later. The subsequent cut becomes longer and more aggressive, placing increasing strain on recovery and performance. Each cycle raises the cost of the next one, even though the physique rarely improves in proportion to the effort invested.

The outcome is predictable:

- Strength declines

- Recovery erodes

- Muscle mass is lost

- The physique briefly looks leaner—then rebounds

For adults with limited recovery capacity, this cycle is inefficient at best and destructive at worst.

The Scale Weight Obsession

One of the most common reasons fat loss fails is an overreliance on scale weight as the primary measure of progress. The scale provides a single number, but no context. Day-to-day decisions are often made off a number that reflects hydration, digestion, and sodium more than fat or muscle. It tells you that weight has changed, not why.

It cannot distinguish between fat loss, muscle loss, water shifts, or glycogen depletion. Each of these can move the scale independently of meaningful body composition change. As a result, scale weight often reflects short-term physiology rather than real progress.

A lifter can lose ten pounds and look worse—smaller, flatter, weaker. Another can remain the same body weight and look dramatically better. The difference isn't the number; it's tissue quality.

Despite this, most decisions are made in reaction to a single morning weigh-in. A routine meant to guide progress quietly turns into a daily referendum on whether the plan is "working." When weight stalls, calories are cut further. Cardio is added indiscriminately. Carbohydrates are removed without cause. Performance signals are dismissed.

This reactive approach slowly erodes the very tissue responsible for a lean, capable physique. When strength is collapsing, energy is depleted, and training feels like survival, the strategy is broken—regardless of what the scale reports.

Electronic scales worsen this problem by creating a false sense of precision. Decimals—0.2 pounds up, 0.4 pounds down—suggest accuracy and meaning that simply isn't there. Day-to-day body weight can fluctuate by several pounds due to hydration, sodium, carbohydrate intake, glycogen levels, digestion, inflammation, and sleep. The scale records all of it as if it were success or failure.

This encourages overreaction. A minor increase becomes a reason to tighten restriction. A brief drop becomes justification to push harder. The scale turns into a feedback loop that rewards emotional decisions instead of strategic ones.

The issue isn't the device, it's how it's used. Scales are useful for identifying long-term trends, not issuing daily verdicts. Used properly, the scale is a blunt reference tool. Used obsessively, it becomes a source of anxiety that drives poor decisions and worse outcomes.

Muscle Loss: The Hidden Cost of Dieting

Muscle is metabolically expensive tissue. It requires ongoing energy not just to build, but to maintain—fuel for repair, neural signaling, and readiness to perform. When calories drop too low, protein intake is insufficient, or training stress exceeds recovery capacity, the body looks for efficiencies. Muscle, from a survival standpoint, is optional. Reducing it lowers daily energy demands.

This is why muscle loss during dieting isn't a rare accident, it's a predictable outcome when constraints are too aggressive. In a steep calorie deficit, muscle protein breakdown increases while muscle protein synthesis becomes harder to stimulate. If resistance training quality declines or protein intake is inadequate, the signal to preserve muscle weakens further. The body responds rationally by shedding tissue it no longer sees as necessary.

What follows is a vicious cycle. An aggressive diet produces rapid weight loss, but some of that loss comes from lean mass. As muscle is lost, resting energy expenditure drops and spontaneous activity often declines as well. The metabolism hasn't been "damaged"—it has adapted to a smaller, less costly body.

When the diet ends, fat regain becomes easier. Appetite rebounds faster than energy expenditure, training performance is slower to recover, and the body preferentially restores fat rather than muscle. The next fat-loss attempt now starts from a worse position: less muscle, lower calorie tolerance, and reduced performance capacity. To see progress again, the lifter cuts harder—restarting the cycle.

Over time, this pattern quietly degrades body composition. The scale may trend downward across years, but the physique underneath becomes smaller, softer, and less capable. Strength is harder to regain. Dieting feels more punishing. Results become less durable.

Many lifters don't fail because they lack discipline. They fail because they repeatedly apply strategies that trade muscle for speed. Without prioritizing muscle retention—through adequate protein, intelligent deficits, and recoverable training—fat loss becomes progressively harder, not easier.

The Problem Isn't Effort — It's Strategy

Most people don't fail because they don't try hard enough. They fail because they followed advice designed for:

- Bodybuilders peaking for competition

- Enhanced athletes

- Influencers selling extremes

Body recomposition exists specifically to solve this problem.

Chapter 2
What Body Recomposition Actually Is

Body recomposition is often dismissed as something that only happens to beginners or as a vague promise that sounds good but rarely delivers. Both views miss the point. Recomposition is not luck, novelty, or a loophole in physiology—it is a predictable outcome when the body is given clear priorities and sufficient resources.

At its core, body recomposition is the simultaneous reduction of body fat and the maintenance—or gradual increase—of lean muscle mass. The goal is not rapid weight loss or dramatic weekly scale changes. In fact, the scale often moves very little. Recomposition is about improving tissue quality: less fat, more or better-preserved muscle, and a physique that looks and performs differently even when body weight remains stable.

Fat loss during recomposition is governed by energy balance. A calorie deficit must exist, but it does not need to be extreme. Muscle retention, on the other hand, is driven by a separate set of signals. Resistance training provides mechanical tension that tells the body muscle tissue is still required. Protein intake supplies the amino acids necessary to repair and maintain that tissue. Recovery—through sleep, stress management, and appropriate training volume—determines whether the body can respond to those signals effectively.

When these inputs align, the body can use stored fat to help meet energy demands while allocating incoming nutrients toward muscle repair and maintenance. This is not a violation of energy balance. It is a matter of nutrient partitioning—directing limited resources toward preserving lean mass rather than sacrificing it for speed.

Recomposition is most likely when the calorie deficit is small to moderate, training quality remains high, and recovery demands do not exceed capacity. As deficits become more aggressive, training stress increases, or recovery deteriorates, the body shifts priorities away from muscle preservation. At that point, recomposition gives way to simple weight loss, often at the expense of lean mass.

Certain populations experience recomposition more easily. Beginners and returning lifters benefit from heightened sensitivity to training stimuli. Individuals with higher body fat have greater stored energy available to support muscle maintenance. Adults who are organizing their training, nutrition, and recovery more intelligently for the first time often see rapid improvements in body composition without extreme measures.

Intermediate lifters can still recompose, but the margin for error is narrower. Small mistakes in calorie intake, protein consumption, training volume, or recovery add up faster. Progress tends to be slower and more subtle, requiring patience and restraint rather than constant adjustment.

This leads to the central challenge of recomposition: time horizon. Recomposition rewards consistency, stable habits, and performance-focused training. It punishes plan-hopping, scale obsession, and short-term thinking. Because muscle is being preserved, fat loss appears slower on the scale. Because progress is gradual, it's easy to doubt the process.

But fat loss that preserves muscle is inherently slower—and far more durable. Recomposition builds a physique that lasts because it improves the foundation rather than eroding it. The tradeoff is patience. The payoff is permanence.

Chapter 3
Energy Balance Without the Myths

Yes, fat loss requires a calorie deficit. That principle is non-negotiable. But reducing fat loss to "eat less" misses the more important question: how that deficit is created and how large it is. Two deficits with the same weekly calorie reduction can produce very different outcomes depending on what the body is being asked to sacrifice in the process.

A large deficit created through severe food restriction is not equivalent to a smaller deficit supported by resistance training, adequate protein, and recoverable stress. A 1,000-calorie deficit achieved through starvation prioritizes speed at the expense of lean mass, performance, and long-term adherence. A 300-calorie deficit created while training hard and eating enough protein preserves muscle, maintains output, and produces fat loss that doesn't immediately unravel.

When calories drop, the body responds predictably. Non-exercise activity decreases without conscious awareness. Resting energy expenditure declines as the body becomes more efficient. Hunger increases to drive intake back up. Training output drops as available energy narrows. These responses are often labeled as "metabolic damage," but that framing is inaccurate. The body isn't broken; it's protecting itself.

These adaptations are normal and expected. What changes is the speed and severity with which they appear. Aggressive dieting accelerates every one of these responses. The larger the deficit, the faster the body pulls back on expenditure and pushes harder on hunger, making continued progress increasingly costly.

For recomposition, smaller deficits consistently outperform aggressive ones. The goal is not maximum weight loss—it is maximum muscle retention alongside steady fat loss. High-quality training must remain possible, recovery must remain manageable, and performance must stay relatively stable. Strength retention becomes the clearest indicator that muscle is being preserved. When loads and repetitions are holding, the signal to keep muscle remains strong.

When deficits become too aggressive, the warning signs appear quickly. Feeling cold, weak, mentally preoccupied with food, and stalled despite further calorie reductions is not a failure of discipline. It is a sign that the body is under-fueled and pushing back. At that point, more restriction doesn't create progress—it deepens the problem.

Recomposition succeeds by working with biology, not against it. Respecting energy balance means accepting that slower, controlled deficits produce better body composition, more reliable performance, and results that last beyond the diet itself.

Part I — Key Takeaways

- Bulk/cut cycles fail most natural lifters

- Scale weight alone is misleading

- Muscle loss is the hidden cost of aggressive dieting

- Recomposition prioritizes muscle retention first

- Small, intelligent deficits outperform extremes

Part II

Body recomposition does not require dietary extremes. It requires correct priorities.

Most nutrition plans fail not because calories were wrong, but because macronutrients were mismanaged — protein too low, carbohydrates treated as optional, dietary fat quietly consuming the entire calorie budget.

This section establishes a clear hierarchy: what matters most, what supports it, and what must be constrained.

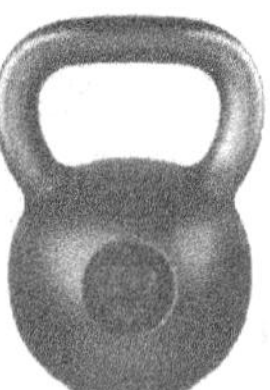

Chapter 4
Protein-The Non Negotiable

If body recomposition had a hierarchy, protein would sit alone at the top. No other nutritional variable comes close in importance for preserving—and in some cases building—muscle while losing fat.

Why Protein Matters More During Fat Loss

Resistance training provides the signal for muscle retention. It tells the body, "this tissue is still required." Protein provides the raw materials to meet that demand—amino acids to repair damage, rebuild structure, and maintain lean mass. Remove either one and the message collapses: without training, the body has no reason to hold muscle; without protein, it has no resources to do so.

During a calorie deficit, the environment becomes inherently more catabolic. The body is trying to conserve energy, so muscle protein breakdown rises and muscle protein synthesis becomes harder to stimulate. In plain terms: it becomes easier to lose muscle and harder to build or even maintain it. The body isn't thinking about physique goals, it's prioritizing survival and efficiency, and muscle is expensive tissue.

Higher protein intake shifts that balance in your favor. It reduces the net loss of muscle by lowering breakdown and supporting synthesis when training provides the stimulus. It also increases satiety, which makes adherence easier—because the best plan is the one you can execute consistently. And because lean mass is a major contributor to resting energy expenditure, preserving muscle helps preserve resting metabolic rate, making future dieting less punishing.

This isn't edgy or debatable. It's one of the most consistently supported conclusions in nutrition and resistance training research: if you want to lose fat without shrinking, resistance training and adequate protein are the non-negotiables.

How Much Protein Is Enough?

Protein needs increase as calories decrease.

Evidence-based targets for recomposition:

- 0.7–1.0 g per pound of lean body mass, or

- 0.6–0.8 g per pound of bodyweight for most lifters

Leaner individuals, aggressive dieters, and those training hard benefit from the higher end of the range.

If fat loss is the goal, err on the side of more protein—not less.

Is "Too Much Protein" a Problem?

For healthy individuals, there is no credible evidence that higher protein intake damages kidney function or bone health. These concerns stem largely from outdated hypotheses and clinical observations in populations with pre-existing kidney disease—not from data on resistance-trained, healthy adults. In lifters, higher protein intakes are consistently shown to be safe, well tolerated, and beneficial for body composition.

Concerns about protein and kidney damage are primarily based on observations in people with existing kidney disease. In this population, higher protein intake can worsen kidney function, because damaged kidneys struggle to cope with the increased nitrogenous waste load, potentially accelerating disease progression. That's why protein restriction is often recommended in chronic kidney disease management.

What is real are diminishing returns. Once protein intake reaches a level sufficient to maximize muscle retention and support recovery, additional protein does not continue to improve outcomes. Muscle protein synthesis plateaus, and further increases simply replace other calories rather than enhancing results.

This introduces a meaningful opportunity cost. Calories are finite, especially during fat loss. When protein intake becomes excessively high, it often crowds out carbohydrates and fats that serve critical roles. Carbohydrates support training intensity, volume tolerance, and recovery. Dietary fats support hormonal function, satiety, and long-term adherence. Undermining either in the name of "more protein" can quietly degrade performance and sustainability—even while protein intake looks optimal on paper.

The objective, then, is not maximal protein intake, but adequate protein intake. Enough to clearly protect lean mass, support recovery, and preserve strength—while still allowing room for carbohydrates that fuel training and fats that support health and adherence. Protein should anchor the diet, not dominate it.

At the same time, the risks are not symmetrical. Excess protein may be inefficient, but insufficient protein during fat loss is reliably destructive. In a calorie deficit, low protein intake accelerates muscle protein breakdown, reduces recovery capacity, and leads to strength loss. Weight may still decrease, but a disproportionate share comes from lean tissue, resulting in a smaller, weaker physique.

Over time, this tradeoff compounds. Each diet cycle performed with inadequate protein leaves the lifter with less muscle, a lower calorie tolerance, and poorer training capacity. Fat loss becomes harder, not easier. What begins as a "successful" diet often ends as a long-term setback.

In practical terms, excess protein wastes some calories. Inadequate protein wastes muscle. During fat loss, that distinction determines whether progress is temporary—or durable.

Protein Distribution

Total daily protein intake matters most. Distribution is secondary.

That said:

- 3–5 protein-rich meals per day

- 25–40 g protein per meal

This improves muscle protein synthesis across the day and supports satiety. Progress comes from repeating the essentials, not executing them flawlessly.

Animal vs. Plant Protein

Animal and plant proteins can both support muscle maintenance and growth, but they differ in efficiency and planning requirements.

Animal proteins generally provide complete amino acid profiles, meaning they contain all essential amino acids in sufficient proportions to stimulate muscle protein synthesis. They also tend to be higher in leucine, the key amino acid that helps trigger the muscle-building process, and are more bioavailable—digested and utilized more efficiently by the body. This makes it easier to meet protein needs with fewer total calories and less planning.

Plant proteins can still work for lifters, but they usually require higher total intake to achieve the same effect. Many plant protein sources are lower in one or more essential amino acids and have less leucine per serving. Combining different plant sources—such as legumes with grains—helps improve amino acid completeness. Plant proteins also often come packaged with more carbohydrates or fats, which can be beneficial or limiting depending on overall calorie targets.

Because of these differences, vegetarian or vegan lifters are generally best served by aiming for a slightly higher protein intake—about 10–20% more than omnivorous lifters—and planning meals deliberately. When total intake is sufficient and sources are chosen thoughtfully, plant-based diets can support recomposition, but they leave less margin for error.

Case Study: Protein Neglect vs. Protein Priority
Subject A

- 180 lb male

- ~120 g protein/day

- Aggressive calorie deficit

- Loses 15 lb in 12 weeks

- Significant strength loss

- Appears smaller, not leaner

Subject B

- Same stats

- ~180 g protein/day

- Modest calorie deficit

- Loses 8 lb in 12 weeks

- Strength largely maintained

- Visible muscle definition improves

Two lifters with identical starting points followed different protein strategies. The lower-protein, aggressive deficit produced faster weight loss—but at the cost of strength and muscle, leaving the lifter smaller rather than leaner. The higher-protein, moderate deficit resulted in slower weight loss, preserved strength, and visibly improved muscle definition. Same effort, different priorities—very different outcomes.

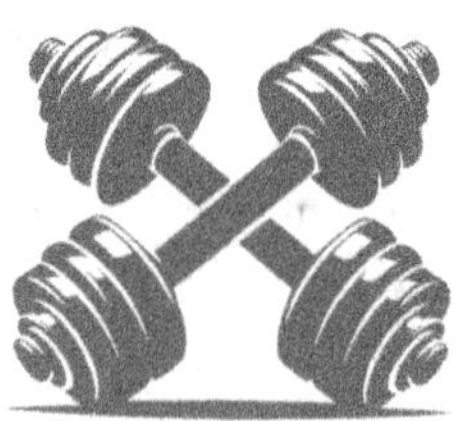

Chapter 5
Carbohydrates—Fuel, Not the Enemy

Carbohydrates have been unfairly blamed for decades, largely because they're easy to vilify and quick to cut. For lifters, that mistake carries a cost. Carbohydrates are not optional; they are performance fuel.

Resistance training relies heavily on glycogen, the stored form of carbohydrate in muscle. When glycogen is adequate, training feels sharp: loads move faster, volume is tolerable, technique holds, and recovery between sessions improves. When carbohydrates are restricted, that fuel tank runs low. Sets feel heavier, work capacity drops, and performance declines—often misinterpreted as age, poor genetics, or "fat loss working."

For lifters pursuing recomposition, performance is the signal that protects muscle. Undermining that signal by under-fueling with carbohydrates weakens training quality and increases the risk of muscle loss. Fat loss that compromises training isn't efficient, it's self-defeating.

Carbohydrates don't prevent fat loss. They enable the kind of training that makes fat loss worth pursuing.

Why Carbs Matter During Recomposition

Carbohydrates play a direct, practical role in lifting performance. They replenish muscle glycogen, support training intensity, reduce perceived effort, and improve recovery between sessions. When carbohydrate intake is adequate, lifters can train harder, maintain volume, and execute movements with consistency.

Low-carb dieting while lifting often produces the opposite effect. Training volume drops, pumps disappear, technique degrades, and strength slowly regresses. These changes are frequently misinterpreted as signs that fat loss is "working," when they are actually signs of under-fueling.

Fat loss that degrades training quality undermines recomposition. When performance erodes, the signal to retain muscle weakens—making the outcome slower, harder, and less durable.

Glycogen Fuels Lifting — Not Fat

Resistance training relies heavily on glycogen—the stored form of carbohydrate in muscle—to fuel repeated, high-intensity efforts. While fat can support low-intensity activity, lifting weights depends on glycogen to sustain load, volume, and technical precision.

When glycogen is low, the effects are immediate and predictable. Sets feel heavier than they should. Volume tolerance drops as fatigue accumulates faster. Technique degrades because the nervous system and musculature can't sustain quality output under load. None of this reflects progress, it reflects a fuel shortage.

Strength loss is not proof that fat loss is working. It is often proof that training is being under-fueled. When performance declines, the body receives a weaker signal to retain muscle, increasing the risk that weight loss comes from the wrong tissue.

Good Carbs or Bad Carbs?

The distinction between "good" and "bad" carbohydrates is largely an oversimplification. Carbohydrates aren't moral, and they aren't inherently harmful or beneficial on their own. What matters—especially for lifters—is context, form, and quantity.

Carbohydrates that are minimally processed, higher in fiber, and more nutrient-dense tend to be easier to manage during fat loss. Foods like rice, potatoes, oats, beans, and whole grains reliably replenish muscle glycogen while also supporting satiety, digestion, and overall diet quality. They're predictable, filling, and compatible with long-term consistency.

Highly processed carbohydrates, on the other hand, are easier to overconsume. Sugary snacks, refined baked goods, and liquid sugars provide calories quickly but do little to control appetite or improve training performance. They aren't inherently toxic, but they are less useful when the goal is recomposition.

The real distinction isn't good versus bad—it's useful versus unhelpful. Carbohydrates that support training quality, recovery, and appetite control make fat loss easier and more sustainable. Those that add calories without improving performance make it harder to stay on track.

A small amount of refined carbohydrates—especially around training—can fit without issue. Problems arise when they dominate the diet. For recomposition, the most effective carbohydrates are the ones that fuel hard training and support consistency over time.

How Many Carbs Should You Eat?

Carbohydrate needs are not fixed. They depend on how much you train, how often you train, and how well you personally tolerate carbohydrates. Higher training volume and frequency increase glycogen demand, while individual tolerance determines how many carbohydrates can be consumed comfortably without disrupting appetite, digestion, or adherence.

General recomposition ranges:

- 0.75–1.25 g carbs per lb bodyweight for moderate training

- Up to ~1.5–2.0 g per lb for higher-volume lifters

During recomposition, protein stays high to protect muscle and support recovery. Dietary fat remains adequate to maintain hormonal function and adherence. Carbohydrates become the primary adjustment lever—scaled up or down to match training demands and create the desired calorie balance without compromising performance.

Carb Timing

Nutrient timing does not override total intake, but it can meaningfully improve training quality. Placing carbohydrates around training helps ensure adequate energy before a session and supports glycogen replenishment and recovery afterward.

This does not require rigid rules or a rushed post-workout shake. The narrow "anabolic window" is largely a myth. What matters more is that training is fueled and total daily intake is appropriate.

The "anabolic window" refers to the idea that there is a very short period—often said to be 30–60 minutes after training—during which you must consume protein (and carbs) or you'll miss your chance to build muscle.

That idea is largely outdated.

Resistance training increases muscle protein synthesis for many hours after a workout—often 24 hours or more. As long as total daily protein and calories are adequate, muscle growth does not hinge on hitting a narrow post-workout deadline.

Post-workout nutrition can still be useful, especially if:

- You trained fasted

- Your last meal was several hours earlier

- You're training again later the same day

But it's not urgent. Missing a shake doesn't cost you muscle.

The practical takeaway:

Totals matter most. Timing can help. Panic is unnecessary.

For most lifters, training fed—rather than fasted—leads to better performance, higher-quality sessions, and more consistent progress.

Common Low-Carb Mistakes

Three common mistakes show up repeatedly when lifters adopt low-carb approaches. First, carbohydrates are often cut before total calories are addressed, reducing training fuel without solving the energy balance problem. Second, early water and glycogen loss is mistaken for fat loss, creating false confidence while performance quietly declines. Third, the resulting drop in strength and work capacity is blamed on age or genetics rather than under-fueling.

Low-carb approaches can work for sedentary fat loss, where performance demands are low. Recomposition is not sedentary. It requires fuel to support training, recovery, and muscle retention—conditions that chronic carbohydrate restriction often undermines.

Case Study: Carb Reintroduction
Female lifter, 145 lb

- Eating ~1,400 kcal

- ~80 g carbs/day

- Strength stalled

- Fat loss plateaued

Adjustment

- Increase carbs to ~160 g

- Calories unchanged

Outcome

- Training performance improves

- Waist measurement decreases over six weeks

A lifter stalled fat loss and strength on very low carbohydrates despite a calorie deficit. Increasing carbohydrates—without increasing calories—restored training performance and restarted fat loss, evidenced by a reduced waist measurement. The added carbs didn't stop progress; they enabled it.

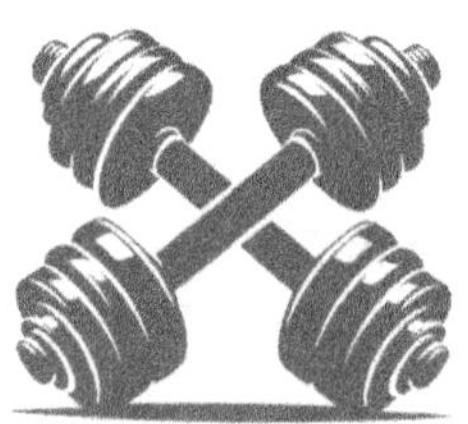

Chapter 6
Dietary Fat—Hormones, Satiety, and Sanity

Dietary fat is often framed as either the enemy or the solution, but neither view is accurate. Fat is best understood as a constraint: it is essential for health and function, yet easy to overconsume and rarely the primary driver of progress in recomposition.

From a physiological standpoint, dietary fat is required for normal hormone production, including testosterone and other steroid hormones that influence recovery, mood, and training readiness. It is also a key component of cell membranes, contributing to cellular integrity and signaling, and it enables the absorption of fat-soluble vitamins (A, D, E, and K), which support immune function, bone health, and overall metabolic health.

Fat also plays a practical role in adherence. Meals that contain some dietary fat tend to be more satisfying and palatable, making it easier to sustain a nutrition plan over time. When fat intake drops too low, hunger often rises and food becomes less enjoyable, increasing the likelihood of overeating later or abandoning the plan altogether.

Extremely low-fat diets can be counterproductive. In addition to increased hunger and reduced satisfaction, chronically low-fat intake may negatively affect testosterone levels and overall hormonal balance, particularly in lifters already under the stress of hard training and a calorie deficit. These effects don't always appear immediately, but over time they can contribute to stalled progress, poor recovery, and declining motivation.

At the same time, fat is calorie dense, providing more than twice the calories per gram as protein or carbohydrates. This makes it easy to overshoot calorie targets without realizing it, especially when fat intake isn't monitored. For this reason, fat should be sufficient—but not excessive. The goal is to meet physiological needs and support adherence while leaving room for protein and carbohydrates, which more directly support muscle retention and training performance.

In recomposition, dietary fat is not a lever to pull aggressively. It is a baseline to respect. Too little undermines health and sustainability; too much crowds out more useful fuel. Keeping fat intake adequate but controlled allows the rest of the system to function as intended.

Minimum Effective Fat Intake

For most lifters:

- 0.25–0.35 g fat per lb bodyweight is sufficient

- Going lower rarely improves fat loss

- Going higher often crowds out carbohydrates

Fat Loss vs. Fat Intake

Eating fat does not make you fat. Body fat gain is driven by sustained calorie surplus, not by any single macronutrient.

However, fat is calorie dense, providing more than twice the calories per gram as protein or carbohydrates. This makes it easy to overconsume without realizing it, especially when portions aren't monitored. For recomposition, fat should be included deliberately—enough to support health and adherence, but not so much that it quietly consumes the calorie budget.

- 1 g fat = 9 calories

- 1 g protein or carbs = 4 calories

This makes fat easy to overconsume unintentionally.

Low-Fat vs. Low-Carb — Which Is Better?

Neither low-fat nor low-carb approaches are universally superior. Their effectiveness depends on context, training demands, and individual response.

Low-fat approaches tend to work better when carbohydrate intake is prioritized to support training performance, hunger remains manageable, and diet structure is consistent enough to control calories without excessive restriction. For lifters training frequently or with higher volume, this approach often preserves performance more reliably.

Low-carb approaches can work better when they noticeably improve appetite control, training volume is moderate rather than high, and simplicity or fewer food decisions improves adherence. In these cases, the reduced carbohydrate intake doesn't meaningfully compromise performance.

For most lifters pursuing recomposition, however, the most reliable solution is a middle ground: moderate dietary fat paired with sufficient carbohydrates. This combination supports training quality, recovery, and adherence without forcing unnecessary trade-offs.

Case Study: Fat Reduction Without Hunger

Male lifter, 200 lb

- ~110 g fat/day

- Struggles to stay in a deficit

Adjustment

- Reduce fat to ~70 g

- Increase carbohydrates

- Calories unchanged

Outcome

- Hunger decreases

- Training performance improves

- Adherence improves

Reducing dietary fat—while keeping calories the same—lowered hunger, improved training performance, and increased adherence. Fat loss didn't require eating less food overall; it required reallocating calories toward more performance-supportive macros.

Chapter 7
Counting Calories vs Counting Macros

Counting calories and counting macronutrients are often framed as opposing strategies. In reality, they answer different questions and operate at different levels of control.

Calories determine whether body weight changes.Macronutrients determine *what* changes.

Understanding the distinction is essential for anyone pursuing body recomposition rather than simple weight loss.

What Counting Calories Actually Controls

Counting calories focuses exclusively on total energy intake. It answers a single question: *How much energy am I consuming?*

From a purely energetic standpoint, this is sufficient to produce weight change. A sustained calorie deficit will result in weight loss. A surplus will result in weight gain. Calories set the direction of change.

What calorie counting does **not** account for is how the body meaningfully responds to that intake. Calories alone do not tell you:

- Whether weight lost is coming from fat or muscle

- Whether training performance is being supported or undermined

- Whether recovery capacity is adequate

- Whether hunger and adherence are sustainable

A 1,800-calorie diet built primarily from low-protein, low-carbohydrate foods will have dramatically different effects than a 1,800-calorie diet structured to support resistance training. Yet calorie counting treats them as equivalent.

For general weight loss, this limitation may be acceptable. For recomposition, it is not.

What Counting Macros Adds

Counting macros does not replace calorie control—it *organizes* it.

By tracking protein, carbohydrates, and fats, you are no longer reacting to a single number. You are deliberately allocating calories toward specific physiological outcomes.

- **Protein** is prioritized to preserve (and sometimes build) lean muscle mass

- **Carbohydrates** are structured to fuel training performance and recovery

- **Dietary fats** are kept sufficient to support hormones, satiety, and long-term adherence

Calories still matter, but they are now constrained within a framework that supports the demands of training and recovery.

Macro tracking transforms calorie control from a blunt instrument into a precision tool.

Why Calories Alone Fall Short for Recomposition

Recomposition requires competing goals to be satisfied simultaneously:

- Fat loss through an energy deficit

- Muscle retention through mechanical tension and protein availability

- Performance preservation through adequate fueling

Calories alone cannot balance these demands. Without macro structure, calorie reduction often leads to:

- Protein being cut unintentionally

- Carbohydrates being reduced below performance-supporting levels

- Dietary fat fluctuating without awareness

The result is a diet that technically "works" for weight loss but fails to support training quality. When performance drops, muscle loss becomes more likely—even if protein intake is adequate on paper.

Two diets with identical calories can produce completely different outcomes depending on macronutrient distribution. One preserves strength and improves body composition. The other produces a smaller, weaker version of the same physique.

Macros as the Mechanism of Control

Macros are not about micromanagement or perfection. They are about directing limited calories toward the variables that matter most.

For recomposition:

- Calories set the **boundary**

- Macros determine the **response**

When protein is anchored, carbohydrates are adjusted around training demands, and fat is kept within a functional range, the body is far more likely to lose fat while preserving muscle.

This is not complexity for its own sake. It is clarity.

When Calorie Counting Alone May Be Enough

There are situations where calorie counting is sufficient:

- Sedentary individuals focused purely on weight loss

- Short-term dieting without performance goals

- Early stages of behavior change where simplicity matters most

As training becomes more demanding and goals become more specific, the limitations of calorie-only approaches become more apparent.

Recomposition is a precision goal. It requires precision inputs.

The Practical Takeaway

Counting macros is not about obsessing over numbers. It is about aligning intake with intent.

If your goal is simply to weigh less, calories may be enough.If your goal is to look, perform, and function better at the same body weight—or while losing slowly—macros matter.

Calories decide *if* change happens.Macros decide *what kind* of change you get.

For recomposition, that distinction makes all the difference.

Part II — Key Takeaways

- Protein is non-negotiable during recomposition

- Carbohydrates protect training quality

- Dietary fat supports hormones and adherence—but must be constrained

- Protein stays high, fats stay adequate, carbs adjust

- Recomposition fails when one macronutrient is ignored

Part III

Training, Recovery, and Calorie Alignment

Body recomposition does not happen through nutrition alone.

Calories and macronutrients only work when paired with the right training signal and sufficient recovery capacity. Without both, the body has no reason to retain metabolically expensive muscle tissue during a calorie deficit.

This section explains how to structure training so the body clearly understands one thing: **Muscle is still required. Fat is not.**

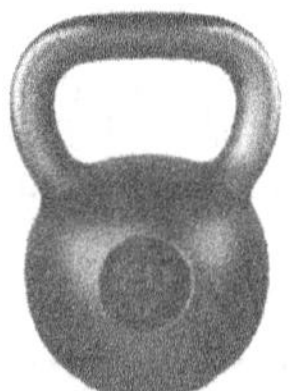

Chapter 8
Recomposition

Recomposition lives in a narrow window. The body must be stressed enough to justify keeping muscle but not so stressed that recovery collapses under a calorie deficit. This is why more training is not better training during recomposition. The limiting factor is not motivation or effort—it is recoverability.

A calorie deficit reduces available energy, hormonal support, and adaptive capacity. Training that ignores this reality quickly becomes self-defeating. Recomposition succeeds when training stress is deliberate, targeted, and sustainable, not maximal.

Maximum Volume for Results (MVR) refers to the highest amount of training volume an individual can perform while still producing positive adaptations. Below MVR, additional work can improve outcomes. Above it, fatigue accumulates faster than recovery, and performance begins to decline. Importantly, MVR is not a fixed number. It shifts based on energy intake, sleep, stress, training age, and current goals. In a calorie surplus, MVR tends to be higher. During fat loss or recomposition, it contracts. Productive training is not about pushing volume as high as possible, but about staying within the range where work remains recoverable and mechanically effective

Volume: How Much Is Enough?

Training volume produces results only within a recoverable range. This range—often described as *maximum volume for results (MVR)*—represents the highest amount of work that meaningfully contributes to adaptation rather than fatigue. Importantly, MVR is not fixed. It shifts based on energy availability, recovery resources, and performance demands.

In a calorie surplus, MVR tends to be higher. Additional volume can sometimes accelerate hypertrophy because fatigue is more easily resolved and loading quality can be maintained. In a calorie deficit, MVR contracts. Recovery capacity is reduced, and the margin between productive volume and excessive fatigue becomes narrower. During recomposition, pushing volume upward often exceeds MVR, while maintaining—or slightly reducing—volume more often keeps training within it.

This distinction matters because muscle retention and growth are driven primarily by mechanical tension delivered with high execution quality. Once volume exceeds MVR, fatigue rises faster than stimulus. Loads drop, technique degrades, and repetitions become less mechanically effective. At that point, adding sets increases stress without strengthening the signal to preserve muscle.

Volume performed beyond MVR is commonly referred to as "junk volume": work that contributes little to adaptation while consuming recovery resources. Research examining volume-response relationships consistently shows diminishing—and eventually negative—returns once recoverable thresholds are exceeded, particularly under conditions of reduced energy intake.

For most lifters, effective recomposition training falls within a moderate-volume range—often around 8–15 challenging reps per muscle group per week. This range reflects where MVR typically sits for trained individuals dieting or recomposing, not a target that must be maximized.

When strength trends downward, soreness lingers, or motivation erodes, the problem is rarely insufficient stimulus. More often, training volume has drifted beyond MVR. In these cases, small volume reductions can restore load stability and execution quality, bringing training back into the productive range.

More volume feels like effort.

Staying within MVR is what produces results.

Intensity and Proximity to Failure

Volume determines how much work you do. Intensity determines whether that work matters.

Training too far from failure fails to create sufficient mechanical tension. The muscle is worked but not challenged. The body perceives this as optional effort and responds accordingly. On the other end of the spectrum, training to failure on every set generates excessive fatigue, reduces performance in subsequent sets and sessions, and inflates recovery cost without increasing stimulus.

For recomposition, the most effective balance lies in 1–3 reps in reserve (RIR) for most working sets. This range provides enough tension to maintain strength and muscle while preserving recovery. Sets feel hard, but not destructive. Performance can be repeated week to week.

Failure has a place—but it must be used intentionally. It is best reserved for isolation movements, final sets, or phases where recovery is robust. When failure becomes habitual, strength erodes and the training signal degrades.

The priority during recomposition is not novelty or sensation. It is strength retention. If loads are holding steady and execution remains solid, the body has a reason to keep muscle. If loads are slipping because fatigue has overtaken tension, muscle becomes expendable.

Training Frequency

Training frequency determines how that volume and intensity are distributed.

For recomposition, training a muscle group twice per week consistently outperforms once-weekly splits. Higher frequency allows volume to be spread across sessions, reducing per-session fatigue and improving stimulus quality. Technique stays sharper, loads feel more manageable, and recovery between sessions improves.

This does not require more exercises or complicated programming. In fact, simplicity is often an advantage. Repeating key movements more frequently reinforces skill, improves efficiency, and strengthens the neural component of strength—an often-overlooked factor in muscle retention.

Higher frequency also creates more frequent reminders to the body that muscle is required. Instead of one exhaustive session followed by long recovery, the signal is refreshed regularly without overwhelming recovery capacity.

You do not need more exercises.

You need better execution, repeated across the week.

The Core Principle

Recomposition training is not about doing everything you can tolerate. It is about doing what you can recover from consistently. Volume must be sufficient but restrained. Intensity must be high enough to demand strength, but not so high that it sabotages future sessions. Frequency must distribute stress intelligently, not multiply it.

When volume, intensity, and frequency are balanced, training sends a clear, repeated message: this muscle is still necessary. When they are mismanaged, fatigue replaces tension, and muscle becomes a liability the body is eager to shed.

Recomposition rewards restraint, precision, and patience.

It punishes excess—even when that excess looks like effort.

Training Is the Signal

Nutrition determines what the body *can* do—it sets the ceiling for energy availability, recovery, and adaptation. Training determines what the body *must* do—it tells the body which tissues are required to meet those demands.

If resistance training does not provide a clear, ongoing signal that strength and muscle are necessary, the body has no reason to preserve them during fat loss. Weight may still come down, but the loss will include muscle alongside fat.

This is why many lifters get lighter without getting better. The scale moves, but performance declines, physiques flatten, and the outcome is a smaller, weaker version of the same body rather than meaningful improvement.

Mechanical Tension Is the Primary Driver

Muscle retention and growth are driven primarily by **mechanical tension**, not by exhaustion, soreness, or how drained a workout feels. The body does not respond to discomfort—it responds to demand. When muscle is required to produce high levels of force under load, the body has a clear reason to maintain and adapt that tissue.

Mechanical tension is created through the combination of challenging loads, controlled execution, and sufficient proximity to failure. Loads must be heavy enough to require meaningful force production. Repetitions must be controlled so the target muscle, not momentum, bears that load. And sets must be taken close enough to failure that the body perceives the work as demanding. Without these elements, tension is diluted, even if the workout feels exhausting.

This is why volume, variety, and novelty matter far less than most lifters believe. High volume without tension produces fatigue, not adaptation. Constantly rotating exercises may feel productive, but it often prevents progressive overload and weakens the training signal. Novelty can create soreness, but soreness is not a reliable indicator of effective stimulus.

For recomposition, this distinction becomes critical. In a calorie deficit, the body is already looking for ways to conserve energy. If training fails to clearly demand strength, muscle becomes an obvious target for reduction. The goal is not to annihilate the muscle with endless sets or metabolic circuits. The goal is to repeatedly demonstrate that the muscle is still required for survival and performance.

Effective recomposition training prioritizes maintaining load, preserving execution quality, and keeping effort high enough to maintain strength. When strength is stable, the signal to retain muscle remains strong. When strength declines because tension has been replaced with fatigue, the signal weakens—and muscle loss follows.

If training does not demand strength, the body will not maintain it. Mechanical tension is the language muscle understands, and during fat loss, it must be spoken clearly and consistently.

Rest Periods and MVR

Rest periods determine whether training volume stays within MVR or quietly exceeds it. When rest is too short, fatigue accumulates faster than recovery, force output drops, and execution degrades. The workload may look the same on paper, but the mechanical signal weakens while recovery cost rises—effectively pushing volume beyond MVR.

For most compound lifts, 2–4 minutes of rest allows sufficient recovery to repeat demanding sets with stable loads and controlled execution. This preserves mechanical tension across sets and keeps volume productive rather than fatiguing.

For isolation movements, 60–120 seconds is typically sufficient. These exercises create less systemic fatigue and recover more quickly. Longer rest rarely improves stimulus; shorter rest is acceptable only if load and execution remain consistent.

Rest should scale with intent:

Heavier loads   and closer proximity to failure require longer rest

Higher reps and   smaller muscle groups require less

The guiding rule is simple: rest long enough to repeat the next set without meaningful loss of load or control. When rest is inadequate, volume drifts past MVR even if set and rep counts stay unchanged.

Short rest does not increase fat loss.
It increases fatigue.

During recomposition, resting longer protects training quality, recovery, and the signal to preserve muscle.

Why "Fat-Burning" Training Fails Lifters

High-rep circuits, constant conditioning, and metabolic-style workouts are often marketed as superior tools for fat loss because they feel demanding. Heart rate stays elevated, sweat pours, and fatigue is immediate. That visible effort is convincing—but it's also misleading.

In practice, these approaches dilute the very signal that preserves muscle. Mechanical tension is reduced when loads are light, rest periods are short, and movements are rushed. Muscles are worked but not *challenged*. The body learns it must tolerate discomfort, not produce force. From a survival perspective, that distinction matters.

At the same time, these methods significantly increase recovery demands. High-volume conditioning creates systemic fatigue that competes with strength training for recovery resources. Joints, connective tissue, and the nervous system absorb repeated stress, often without providing a proportional adaptive benefit. In a calorie deficit—where recovery capacity is already limited—this becomes especially costly.

The result is a resource conflict. Energy, recovery, and adaptive capacity are finite. When they're spent chasing calorie burn through conditioning, less remains to support high-quality strength training. Strength stagnates or declines, training quality erodes, and the signal to preserve muscle weakens.

This is why many lifters lose weight but not muscle selectively. Fat loss does not require special exercises, circuits, or constant exhaustion. It requires an energy deficit. Muscle retention, however, requires a clear and repeated demand for strength. That demand comes from mechanical tension—not metabolic stress.

Training that leaves you exhausted but weaker sends the wrong message. It tells the body that endurance matters more than force, and efficiency matters more than muscle. The scale may move, but the outcome is often a flatter, weaker physique rather than a leaner, more capable one.

Effective recomposition training prioritizes strength first. Conditioning is a tool, not a centerpiece. When fatigue replaces tension as the primary driver of training, fat loss may still occur—but muscle loss is far more likely to come with it.

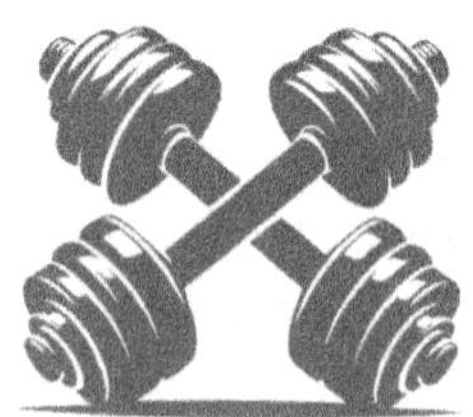

Chapter 9
Recovery Is Not Optional

Recovery is not something you earn by training hard or "deserve" after suffering enough. It is a requirement. Adaptation only occurs when stress is followed by adequate recovery. Without it, training becomes noise—effort expended without progress.

In a calorie deficit, recovery capacity is already reduced. Energy availability is lower, hormonal support is diminished, and the margin for error is smaller. Ignoring this reality doesn't make you disciplined—it guarantees stagnation. The body cannot be trained into adaptation when it lacks the resources to respond.

Sleep: The Primary Recovery Tool

Sleep is the foundation everything else rests on. Training, nutrition, and supplementation all depend on it, and none can compensate when it's missing. For recomposition in particular—where the goal is to lose fat without sacrificing muscle—sleep is not a supporting variable. It is a primary driver.

Physiologically, sleep is when recovery actually happens. Muscle protein synthesis is elevated, tissue repair occurs, and the nervous system resets. Hormones that regulate growth, appetite, and stress are restored toward baseline. When sleep is consistently inadequate, these processes are impaired no matter how well training and nutrition are structured.

Sleep directly affects hormonal regulation. Chronic sleep restriction lowers testosterone and growth hormone while elevating cortisol. This shifts the body toward muscle breakdown and fat storage—exactly the opposite of what recomposition requires. At the same time, insulin sensitivity declines, making nutrient partitioning worse. Calories that might have supported training and recovery are more likely to be stored as fat.

When Sleep Won't Come: Insomnia and Recomposition

Insomnia deserves specific acknowledgment because it is not the same problem as poor sleep habits. Someone who scrolls their phone until midnight and sleeps badly has a behavior problem. Someone with chronic insomnia may do everything right — consistent schedule, dark room, no caffeine after noon, no screens before bed — and still lie awake at two in the morning staring at the ceiling.

The distinction matters because the advice is different. Standard sleep hygiene recommendations, while valid, do not resolve clinical insomnia and can actually increase anxiety in people who are already hyperaware of their sleep. If insomnia is chronic, persistent, and unresponsive to behavioral changes, it warrants conversation with a physician rather than another supplement or another protocol. Cognitive Behavioral Therapy for Insomnia — CBT-I — has the strongest evidence base of any insomnia treatment, including medication, and is worth pursuing seriously.

In the meantime, the recomposition response to poor sleep is not to push harder. It is to reduce training volume modestly, protect protein intake, and extend the timeline. The body cannot be disciplined into recovering from sleep it did not get. Acknowledging that is not weakness — it is accuracy.

Hydration – How Much Is Enough—and Why Water Alone Isn't the Answer

Hydration is not determined by water intake alone. It reflects the body's ability to retain and utilize fluid within tissues, particularly muscle. That process depends on total fluid intake, electrolyte availability, carbohydrate status, and renal regulation—not on how many glasses of water are consumed.

Because of this, there is no single intake target that guarantees adequate hydration. Fluid needs vary with body size, training volume, sweat rate, climate, diet composition, and sodium intake. For recomposition, the relevant question is not *how much water you drink*, but whether hydration is sufficient to support performance, recovery, and stable training output.

That said, practical lower bounds exist. For most lifters, baseline hydration is typically adequate when daily fluid intake falls roughly in the range of 0.5–0.7 ounces of fluid per pound of bodyweight per day, inclusive of all non-alcoholic beverages. Larger lifters, those training frequently, sweating heavily, or consuming higher protein and carbohydrate intakes often require more. During fat loss and recomposition, hydration needs often increase rather than decrease, as reduced glycogen lowers total body water and calorie restriction reduces incidental fluid intake from food.

Electrolytes—particularly sodium—determine whether consumed fluid is retained or rapidly excreted. When sodium intake is too low, hydration status can worsen despite high fluid intake. Frequent urination, flat muscles, early fatigue, and poor pumps are common signs. These effects are especially pronounced in lifters who eat "clean," sweat regularly, and intentionally drink large volumes of plain water.

Carbohydrates matter as well. Muscle glycogen binds water inside the muscle cell. When carbohydrate intake is reduced, glycogen and intracellular water decline together, lowering training capacity even if bodyweight is dropping. Adequate carbohydrate intake supports intracellular hydration, force production, and work capacity during resistance training.

Because hydration fluctuates day to day, sufficiency is best judged through functional indicators rather than exact volumes:

Training performance is stable across sessions

Loads do not feel artificially heavy early in workouts

Soreness resolves predictably between sessions

Urine is pale yellow most of the day

When these conditions are met, hydration is likely sufficient—even if daily intake varies.

The most common hydration mistake among lifters is not drinking too little overall, but failing to scale hydration with training demand while simultaneously restricting sodium or carbohydrates. In these cases, hydration becomes a hidden recovery constraint that lowers effective MVR and distorts performance signals.

Hydration does not need to be optimized obsessively. It needs to be adequate enough that it does not interfere with training quality or recovery. When hydration is sufficient, volume and intensity decisions can be interpreted accurately. When it is not, lifters often change the wrong variables.

Hydration is not just water. It is water, sodium, fuel, and context working together.

HUNGER HORMONES

Ghrelin and leptin are the two primary hormones that regulate hunger and satiety, and they play a central role in why fat loss feels easy at times and brutally difficult at others—especially during recomposition.

Ghrelin is often called the hunger hormone. It is produced primarily in the stomach and rises when the body perceives an energy shortage. Ghrelin signals the brain that it's time to eat, increases appetite, and heightens the reward value of food. When ghrelin is elevated, food is more tempting, portions feel less satisfying, and restraint requires more conscious effort.

Leptin works in the opposite direction. It is produced by fat cells and signals energy sufficiency. When leptin levels are adequate, appetite is suppressed, energy expenditure is supported, and the body is comfortable maintaining its current weight. Leptin essentially tells the brain, "we have enough."

During fat loss—and especially during aggressive dieting—this balance is disrupted. As body fat decreases and calories drop, leptin levels fall while ghrelin levels rise. The brain interprets this combination as a threat to survival. Hunger intensifies, food focus increases, and energy expenditure subtly declines. This isn't a lack of discipline—it's a coordinated biological response.

Sleep plays a critical role in this system. Even short-term sleep deprivation increases ghrelin and decreases leptin, independent of calorie intake. In practical terms, poor sleep makes you hungrier and less satisfied by the same amount of food. Cravings increase, impulse control weakens, and adherence becomes harder—even when calories and macros are unchanged.

This is why hunger during recomposition is not purely a matter of willpower. It is hormonally driven. Large deficits, chronic stress, and poor sleep all push ghrelin higher and leptin lower, making the process feel progressively more difficult over time.

Managing recomposition effectively means respecting this system. Moderate calorie deficits, sufficient protein, adequate carbohydrates, maintenance phases when needed, and consistent sleep all help stabilize leptin and blunt excessive ghrelin signaling. When these hormones are better regulated, hunger becomes manageable, training quality improves, and fat loss becomes sustainable.

In short, ghrelin and leptin don't care about motivation. They respond to energy availability, stress, and sleep. Recomposition succeeds when those signals are managed—not ignored.

Appetite regulation also deteriorates quickly under poor sleep. Hunger hormones become dysregulated: ghrelin increases, leptin decreases, and cravings intensify—especially for highly palatable, calorie-dense foods. What feels like a willpower problem is often a sleep problem. Diet adherence becomes harder not because discipline disappeared, but because biology tilted the playing field.

Training performance suffers as well. Sleep deprivation reduces force output, reaction time, coordination, and pain tolerance. Weights feel heavier, volume tolerance drops, and technique degrades. Over time, this erodes the mechanical tension signal required to preserve muscle. Even if workouts are completed, their quality declines—and quality matters far more than effort.

Recovery between sessions is also compromised. In a calorie deficit, recovery capacity is already limited. Poor sleep further shrinks that capacity, causing fatigue to accumulate across weeks rather than dissipate between workouts. Strength stalls or regresses, soreness lingers, and injury risk rises. These outcomes are often misattributed to age, genetics, or overtraining when sleep is the underlying constraint.

Perhaps most importantly, sleep determines how much stress the body can tolerate. The body does not separate sleep deprivation from training stress or work stress—they all draw from the same recovery pool. When sleep is poor, even moderate training loads can exceed recovery capacity. Managing sleep effectively expands that capacity; neglecting it guarantees friction.

No supplement replaces sleep. No macro strategy overrides it. You cannot "optimize" your way around chronic sleep loss. For recomposition, improving sleep quality often produces faster and more reliable progress than changing calories, macros, or training variables.

In practical terms, consistently getting seven to nine hours of sleep is one of the highest-return investments a lifter can make. It improves performance, preserves muscle, stabilizes appetite, and restores resilience. Sleep doesn't just support recomposition—it makes it possible.

Stress and Allostatic Load

The body does not differentiate between types of stress. Training stress, work stress, emotional stress, and sleep deprivation are processed through the same physiological systems. All of them contribute to what is known as allostatic load—the cumulative burden placed on the body's ability to adapt and recover.

This matters because recovery capacity is finite. When total stress exceeds that capacity, the body shifts from adaptation to conservation. Strength declines, fatigue accumulates, motivation drops, and injury risk rises. These outcomes are often misinterpreted as personal failure or lack of resilience. They are neither.

This is not weakness.It is biology.

During recomposition, managing stress becomes as important as managing calories or training variables. Hard training layered on top of high life stress and poor sleep does not produce faster results—it produces burnout. The body responds to the total demand placed upon it, not just what happens in the gym.

Recovery as a Strategic Variable

Effective recomposition requires treating recovery as a strategic variable, not an afterthought. This means adjusting training volume when sleep is poor, moderating deficits during high-stress periods, and recognizing when maintenance phases are necessary to restore capacity.

Progress does not come from pushing through exhaustion. It comes from applying stress that can be recovered from repeatedly. When recovery is respected, training quality improves, strength stabilizes, and fat loss becomes more predictable.

Recomposition is not about seeing how much you can tolerate.It is about creating conditions where adaptation is possible—and repeatable.

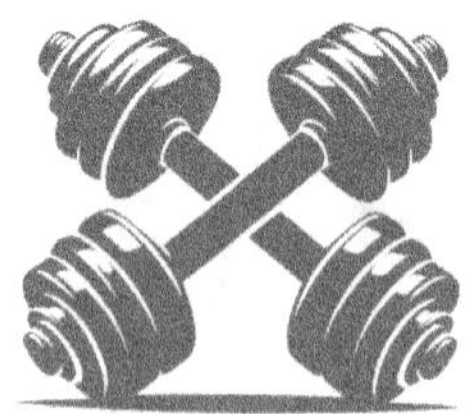

Chapter 10
Cardio—Tool or Saboteur?

Cardio occupies a strange place in fitness culture. It is often treated as either mandatory for fat loss or completely incompatible with strength training. Neither view is accurate. Cardio is a tool—neither inherently good nor inherently harmful. Its value depends entirely on how it is used, how much is applied, and what it is meant to accomplish.

Recomposition does not require cardio, but it can benefit from it when applied intelligently. The mistake most lifters make is assuming that more cardio automatically produces more fat loss. In reality, cardio only contributes to recomposition when it supports training quality, recovery, and adherence rather than competing with them.

When Cardio Helps

Cardio supports recomposition when it improves cardiovascular health and work capacity without compromising strength training. Improved aerobic fitness allows lifters to recover more efficiently between sets and between sessions, reducing perceived effort and fatigue during resistance training. Over time, this can make higher-quality training more sustainable.

Cardio can also help maintain a modest calorie deficit without further restricting food intake. For some lifters, adding a small amount of activity is psychologically easier than eating less. In these cases, cardio functions as a compliance tool rather than a fat-loss driver.

Low-intensity steady-state (LISS) cardio—such as walking, cycling, or incline treadmill work—is generally the most compatible with recomposition. It produces relatively low fatigue, is easy to recover from, and can be performed frequently without interfering with strength training. When cardio is used this way, it complements the overall system rather than disrupting it.

When Cardio Hurts

Cardio becomes counterproductive when it interferes with strength training recovery or replaces resistance training as the primary fat-loss strategy. Excessive cardio increases systemic fatigue, draws from the same recovery pool as lifting, and can blunt strength adaptations—especially in a calorie deficit where recovery capacity is already limited.

Problems also arise when cardio is increased to compensate for poor diet structure. Using cardio to "earn food" or to offset inconsistent eating often leads to a cycle of overexertion and under-recovery. The result is declining performance, rising fatigue, and stalled progress.

High-intensity interval training (HIIT) deserves particular caution. While effective for conditioning, HIIT carries a high recovery cost and overlaps heavily with the stress of resistance training. When layered on top of hard lifting and a calorie deficit, it often accelerates burnout rather than fat loss.

If strength is declining, fatigue is accumulating, and training quality is suffering, cardio is frequently the first variable that should be reduced—not calories. Removing or scaling back cardio often restores performance and allows recomposition to resume without further dietary restriction.

The Right Role for Cardio

In recomposition, cardio should serve strength training, not compete with it. Used sparingly and strategically, it can improve health, support adherence, and modestly increase energy expenditure. Used aggressively or reactively, it undermines recovery and erodes the very muscle recomposition aims to preserve.

Cardio is not a requirement. It is an option. The difference between tool and saboteur lies entirely in how—and why—you use it.

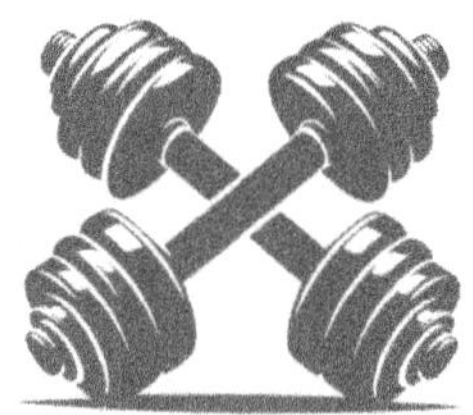

Chapter 11
Aligning Calories With Training Demand

C alories should reflect what the body is being asked to do. Nutrition does not exist in a vacuum—it is meant to support the demands imposed by training. When calorie intake and training demand are misaligned, progress stalls regardless of effort or intent.

Heavy training performed with insufficient fuel creates adaptation resistance. The body receives a strong stimulus to maintain or build muscle, but lacks the energy to respond. Performance stagnates, recovery slows, and fatigue accumulates. The signal is present, but the resources are not. Over time, the body begins to conserve rather than adapt.

The opposite mismatch creates a different problem. Light or inconsistent training paired with excessive calorie intake produces fat gain. Without sufficient demand for those calories, the surplus is stored rather than used for adaptation. In both cases, the issue is not calories alone—it is calories divorced from purpose.

Recomposition succeeds when intake is scaled to match output, allowing the body to meet training demands while maintaining a controlled energy balance.

Training Days vs. Rest Days

Many lifters benefit from modest calorie and carbohydrate cycling across the week. Training days typically warrant higher intake, particularly from carbohydrates, to support performance, glycogen replenishment, and recovery. Rest days, by contrast, often require slightly less fuel, as energy expenditure and recovery demands are lower.

This approach is not metabolic trickery, carb cycling magic, or an attempt to "confuse" the body. It is simple demand matching. Calories are provided when they are most useful and reduced when they are less necessary. The result is better training quality without increasing average weekly intake.

Importantly, the differences between days do not need to be extreme. Small shifts are often sufficient to improve performance and adherence while maintaining a modest weekly deficit.

Maintenance Periods as a Strategy

Maintenance phases are one of the most underused tools in long-term recomposition. Short periods at or near maintenance calories serve a clear physiological and psychological purpose. They restore training performance, reduce adaptive pressure, and allow recovery systems to normalize after prolonged restriction.

Physiologically, maintenance reduces hunger signals, improves hormonal balance, and restores glycogen levels, making future training more productive. Psychologically, it relieves diet fatigue and reinforces the skills required to sustain progress without constant restriction.

Maintenance is not a failure or a loss of discipline. It is a planned reset—a way to consolidate progress rather than sacrifice it. Lifters who use maintenance strategically can extend productive recomposition phases, avoid burnout, and achieve results that last.

Aligning calories with training demand—and knowing when to pause restriction—is not a shortcut. It is how progress is preserved rather than repeatedly undone.

Sample Week: Recomposition in Practice

This example illustrates alignment—not a template.

Subject

- Male lifter, ~180 lb

- Intermediate training age

- Goal: fat loss with strength maintenance

Monday — Upper Body

- Bench Press: 3×5–7 @ 1–2 RIR

- Row Variation: 3×6–8

- Overhead Press: 2×6–8

- Pulldown or Pull-Ups: 3×8–10

- Optional accessories: 2–3 total setsCalories: ~2,600 kcal

Tuesday — Lower Body

- Squat or Leg Press: 3×5–7

- Romanian Deadlift: 3×6–8

- Split Squat or Lunge: 2×8–10

- Leg Curl: 2×10–12Calories: ~2,600 kcal

Wednesday — Rest / Light Cardio

- 30–40 minutes LISSCalories: ~2,300 kcal

Thursday — Upper Body

- Incline or Dumbbell Press: 3×6–8

- Chest-Supported Row: 3×8–10

- Lateral Raise: 3×12–15

- Arm work: 2–4 setsCalories: ~2,600 kcal

Friday — Lower Body
- Deadlift or Hip Thrust: 2–4×4–6

- Front Squat or Hack Squat: 3×6–8

- Hamstring / Calf work: 2–3 sets eachCalories: ~2,600 kcal

Weekend — Rest
- Optional walking or recreational activityCalories: ~2,300–2,400 kcal

Weekly deficit is modest.Training performance is prioritized.Recovery is protected.

Advanced Lifter Warning: Volume Creep

Advanced lifters are especially prone to volume creep—the slow, incremental increase in training volume that occurs when progress becomes harder to perceive. As training age increases, gains arrive more slowly and feedback becomes less obvious. In response, many experienced lifters instinctively add work, assuming that more effort will force adaptation.

In a calorie deficit, this instinct is usually wrong.

Volume creep feels productive because it increases effort and fatigue. Sessions become longer, soreness increases, and the psychological reassurance of "doing more" sets in. But recomposition is not limited by effort—it is limited by recovery. When volume expands beyond recoverable levels, adaptation stalls even as workload increases.

The first thing to erode is load quality. Weights that were once manageable feel heavier. Repetitions slow down. Technique becomes less precise as fatigue accumulates. Mechanical tension—the signal that preserves muscle—declines even though total volume is higher. At the same time, joint and connective tissue stress rises because tissues are being stressed repeatedly without sufficient recovery.

Advanced lifters often mistake these warning signs for a need to push harder. Strength slipping week to week, soreness that lingers across sessions, and declining motivation are interpreted as insufficient effort rather than excessive stress. The result is a feedback loop: more volume produces worse recovery, which produces worse performance, which prompts even more volume.

In recomposition, this loop is destructive.

For experienced lifters, progress depends less on how much work is done and more on how well that work is executed. Fewer sets performed with intent, control, and sufficient load provide a stronger signal than excessive volume performed in a fatigued state. Removing sets often restores performance faster than adding them ever could.

Recovery must also be treated as a limiting factor, not an inconvenience. Sleep quality, stress levels, and calorie availability all cap how much training can be productively absorbed. Ignoring those caps does not build resilience—it degrades it.

During recomposition, the minimum effective dose wins. The goal is not to see how much training you can survive, but how little you need to maintain strength and muscle while fat is lost. For advanced lifters, restraint is not a concession—it is a requirement for continued progress.

Part III — Key Takeaways

- Training is the signal that preserves muscle

- Mechanical tension matters more than fatigue

- Volume must be recoverable in a deficit

- Sleep and stress management are non-negotiable

- Calories must align with training demand

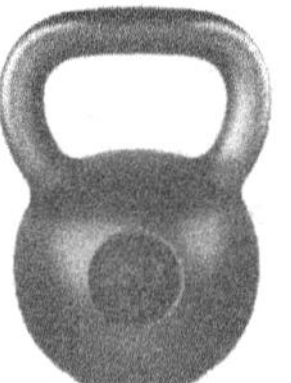

Part IV

Tracking, Adjustments, and Plateaus

Recomposition does not fail because the plan was wrong. It fails because the feedback loop was misunderstood.

Most lifters either track too much and panic—or track too little and drift. Successful recomposition requires learning which signals matter, how long to wait before reacting, and how to adjust without sabotaging long-term results.

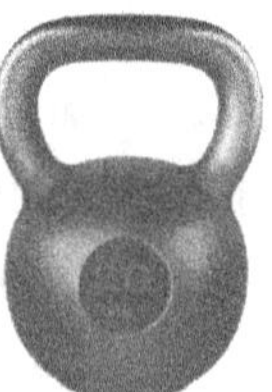

Chapter 12
What to Track (and What to Ignore)

Most people track noise and call it data.

Numbers feel objective, which makes them comforting. But objectivity without context is misleading. Body recomposition produces slow, uneven signals, and when the wrong ones are emphasized, decision-making deteriorates even when execution is consistent.

The scale is the most common example. It reports a single value influenced by hydration, glycogen, sodium, digestion, inflammation, and sleep. Fat loss is only one contributor, and often not the dominant one. Yet the scale is treated as a daily verdict. A small increase creates anxiety. A small decrease creates relief. Neither reflects meaningful change.

Used properly, the scale is not useless—but it is blunt. Its value lies in long-term trends, not daily readings. Weekly averages reveal direction. Individual data points do not. When the scale is used reactively, it stops informing decisions and starts provoking them.

Measurements provide a different signal. Circumference changes reflect tissue redistribution more directly, especially at the waist. A stable bodyweight paired with a shrinking waist is one of the clearest indicators that recomposition is occurring. Fat is being lost while muscle is preserved. This change often appears weeks before the scale acknowledges it.

Performance is the non-negotiable metric. Strength reflects whether the body has sufficient energy and recovery to justify keeping muscle. Stable loads and repetitions under controlled intake signal that the training stimulus remains effective. When strength collapses across multiple sessions, it is rarely a motivation issue. It is feedback that recovery capacity has been exceeded.

The mistake is not tracking too little or too much. It is tracking without hierarchy. When every metric is treated as equally important, the loudest one wins—and that is usually the least reliable.

Effective tracking does not eliminate uncertainty. It teaches restraint in the presence of it. Progress becomes visible only when trends are allowed to form. Interpreting signals too early turns normal variance into self-inflicted disruption.

Chapter 13
The Adjustment Timeline

Most people adjust too fast, not because they are impatient, but because they expect biological change to behave like immediate feedback.

Training sessions provide instant sensation. Food choices produce immediate feelings. Body composition does neither. Fat loss and muscle retention emerge only after enough consistent inputs have accumulated to overwhelm daily noise. When decisions are made before that accumulation occurs, the system is altered before it can respond.

Recomposition amplifies this problem because it operates in narrow margins. Small deficits and recoverable training do not create dramatic shifts. They create slow trends that only appear when allowed to run uninterrupted. Interrupting them resets the process rather than accelerating it.

Short-term signals are especially deceptive. A stable scale can coexist with shrinking measurements. Temporary weight gain can occur alongside fat loss when training stress rises. Strength can feel less stable during phases of adaptation without actually declining. None of these require intervention. All of them punish premature adjustment.

Waiting, in this context, is not passive. It is the discipline of allowing cause and effect to separate. Only when weekly averages stabilize, measurements fail to change, and performance trends flatten does the system provide reliable feedback. Anything earlier is guesswork disguised as decisiveness.

Most recomposition attempts fail not because they were misdesigned, but because they were never given time to reveal whether they worked.

Chapter 14

How to Adjust Without Overcorrecting

When adjustment becomes necessary, the goal is not to create urgency. It is to restore clarity.

Large changes blur feedback. A sharp calorie reduction coinciding with increased cardio and altered training volume produces discomfort quickly, but it also obscures cause and effect. Fatigue rises faster than fat loss. Performance deteriorates before adaptation can occur. The plan becomes harder to execute without becoming more effective.

Effective adjustment respects scale. Small problems require small corrections. A modest reduction in intake, a slight decrease in volume, or the removal of unnecessary stressors preserves the structure that allowed progress to begin in the first place. The system remains recognizable, which makes its response interpretable.

Overcorrection often feels responsible because it creates immediate strain. That strain is mistaken for effort, and effort is mistaken for progress. But recomposition is not driven by suffering. It is driven by sustainable tension applied repeatedly.

The most reliable adjustments preserve training quality. Load is protected. Execution remains sharp. Fatigue is relieved before effort is increased. Only one variable changes at a time, followed by enough time for the body to respond meaningfully.

The difference between successful and failed adjustment is not boldness. It is restraint applied deliberately.

Chapter 15
Plateaus — Real vs. Perceived

Not every stall is a plateau, but most people treat them as if they are.

Weight, measurements, and performance rarely move together. Fat loss can occur without scale change. Strength can stabilize without visual improvement. These mismatches are normal, but they create uncertainty. In that uncertainty, many people assume progress has stopped.

Perceived plateaus are short-lived. They arise from water retention, increased training stress, disrupted sleep, or simple variance. They resolve when consistency continues. Intervening here does not fix a problem—it creates one.

A true plateau is different. It is defined by persistence, not frustration. Weekly weight averages fail to shift. Measurements hold steady. Visual change stalls. Training performance neither improves nor collapses. Nothing is obviously wrong, but nothing is improving.

This distinction is critical because the response must match the reality. Reacting to perceived plateaus increases stress without restoring progress. Responding to true plateaus requires modest, deliberate change designed to reintroduce momentum without dismantling the system.

Patience is the filter that separates the two. Those who wait long enough discover whether progress was merely quiet or genuinely stalled. Those who do not never find out.

Most plateaus are not real. The consequences of misidentifying them are.

Chapter 16
Psychological Traps That Kill Progress

Recomposition does not fail because the plan is wrong. It fails because normal human reactions are misinterpreted as problems that need to be fixed.

Physiologically, the process is straightforward. Apply a small, consistent deficit. Train in a way that preserves strength. Recover well enough to repeat that effort. Over time, body composition improves. Nothing about this is dramatic. And that is precisely why it is difficult to sustain.

Humans are not built to trust slow feedback. When progress is obvious, motivation is easy. When progress becomes quiet, doubt fills the gap. The scale stalls. Mirrors lie. Training feels heavier even when nothing is actually wrong. In that silence, most people assume the plan has stopped working.

It hasn't.

What usually follows is escalation. Calories are cut further. Cardio is added. Training volume creeps upward. Rules tighten. Effort increases, but direction is lost. The system becomes more stressful without becoming more effective. Fatigue accumulates. Performance slips. The very signals that indicate muscle is being preserved begin to degrade.

At this point, many people conclude that recomposition "doesn't work." In reality, it was never allowed to finish.

One of the most common traps is scale fixation. Day-to-day weight fluctuations are interpreted as success or failure, even though they are driven largely by water, glycogen, sodium, digestion, and stress. A single higher weigh-in can undo weeks of patience. A brief drop can justify pushing harder than recovery allows. The scale becomes a trigger rather than a tool.

Comparison is another quiet disruptor. Progress is judged against others—often people with different genetics, recovery capacity, or pharmaceutical support. What looks like discipline elsewhere creates impatience here. The urge to catch up replaces the discipline to stay consistent.

There is also the belief that discomfort is proof of effectiveness. Hunger, exhaustion, and mental strain are treated as signs that the process is "working." When those sensations ease, fear sets in. Eating enough to train well feels like cheating. Rest feels like laziness. Calm is mistaken for complacency.

But recomposition does not reward suffering. It rewards repeatability.

The most destructive trap is panic at normal resistance. Progress always slows as the body adapts. Fat loss becomes less linear. Visual changes take longer to appear. Strength requires more focus to maintain. These are not warnings. They are the expected signs of a system approaching equilibrium. Responding with urgency here does not restore progress—it disrupts it.

Successful recomposition requires emotional restraint more than motivation. The ability to hold steady when feedback is ambiguous. To keep executing when results are subtle. To wait long enough to know whether a change is needed before making one.

Most people do not quit because the process is unbearable. They quit because they stop trusting it. They confuse quiet progress with no progress. They treat patience as passivity and restraint as weakness.

In reality, restraint is the skill being built.

Recomposition works when decisions are made slowly, based on trends rather than moments. When adjustments are deliberate instead of reactive. When discipline is applied to consistency, not escalation.

The body does not require urgency to change. It requires clarity and time.

Those who learn to tolerate the quiet phases are the ones who finish the process.

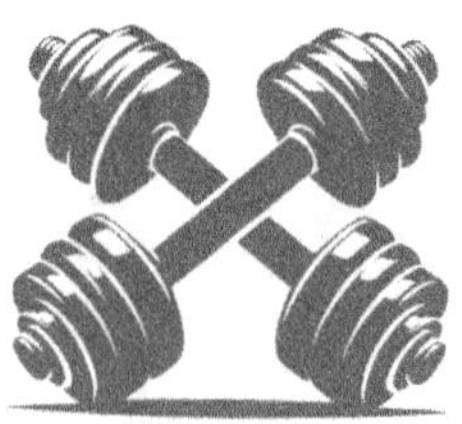

Chapter 17
Maintenance Is Not Quitting

Most physiques are not lost during a diet. They are lost in the weeks that follow it.

Maintenance feels uncomfortable because it removes urgency. There is no immediate target, no visible momentum, no daily confirmation that effort is being rewarded. For people conditioned to equate progress with pressure, this absence feels like drift.

It isn't.

Maintenance is a phase of stabilization, not inactivity. Calories rise enough to restore training performance and recovery without pushing bodyweight upward. Hunger normalizes. Fatigue dissipates. The body stops interpreting intake as a temporary disruption and begins to treat it as safe. This shift matters more than most people realize.

Physiologically, maintenance reduces adaptive pressure. Hormonal signals stabilize. Glycogen is restored. Training output becomes reliable again. These changes are not cosmetic. They determine how effective the next phase will be. Skipping maintenance often means entering the next deficit already depleted.

Psychologically, maintenance exposes fragility. Without restriction, many people fear loss of control. Small increases in bodyweight—often water and glycogen—are interpreted as regression. Panic follows. Calories are cut again. The diet never truly ends, and recovery never fully returns.

This is where most long-term progress is undone.

Maintenance requires a different kind of discipline. Not restraint, but trust. The ability to hold structure without escalation. To eat enough to support training without compensating for it. To tolerate stability without mistaking it for failure.

Done correctly, maintenance consolidates progress. Strength rebounds. Habits become automatic. Food loses emotional charge. The physique becomes easier to sustain because it is no longer defended through constant restriction.

Maintenance is not a pause between "real" phases.It is the phase where results become durable.

Those who skip it remain trapped in cycles of urgency and collapse. Those who learn to live there extend progress without increasing effort. The difference is not willpower. It is timing.

Part IV — Key Takeaways

- Track trends, not days

- Waist measurements often reveal progress first

- Strength retention signals muscle preservation

- Adjust slowly and deliberately

- Maintenance phases are strategic—not failures

Part V

Keeping the Results

Most physiques are not lost during a diet. They are lost after it ends.

Recomposition succeeds or fails based on what happens next—how calories are increased, how training is adjusted, and whether the lifter trusts the process enough to stop "doing more."

This final section explains how to exit recomposition without rebound, how to live at maintenance confidently, and how to avoid restarting the cycle you worked to escape.

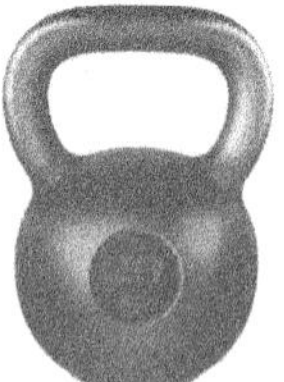

Chapter 18
When Recomposition Is "Done"

Recomposition does not end on a calendar date. The earliest signal is often resistance rather than collapse—progress slows quietly while effort begins to feel heavier than it should.It ends when the body's signals change.

At some point, the same behaviors that once produced fat loss begin to produce friction instead. Progress slows. Recovery tightens. Effort increases without proportional return. This is not a moral failure or a lack of discipline—it is physiology asserting itself.

Recomposition is complete when one or more of the following conditions are met:

- **Fat loss has slowed to a crawl despite consistent execution**

- **Strength and recovery are increasingly difficult to maintain**

- **The desired body composition has been achieved**

Trying to push recomposition indefinitely is a mistake. Past this point, additional restriction produces diminishing returns while extracting a growing recovery and psychological cost. Continued fat loss eventually requires larger deficits, more training stress, or acceptance of performance decline. At that point, the trade-off shifts. What was once productive becomes extractive.

Stopping here is not quitting.It is timing.

Signs You're Ready to Transition

The earliest signal is often anthropometric, not visual. A waist measurement that stabilizes at a lower level—despite continued adherence—usually indicates that most readily accessible fat loss has occurred. Further reductions tend to come slowly and at increasing physiological cost, often without meaningful visual payoff.

Training is the next indicator. Early in recomposition, strength is stable or improving. As energy availability tightens, maintaining numbers begins to feel heavier. Sessions require more psychological effort. Recovery becomes less predictable. This is not weakness—it is a normal response to prolonged constraint.

Hunger and fatigue often rise together. Persistent appetite, poor sleep quality, or low-grade exhaustion are not signs of poor willpower. They are feedback that the system no longer has enough energy to support both adaptation and further loss.

Finally, motivation erodes—not explosively, but quietly. You're still compliant. You're still doing the work. But caring feels harder. This is the early stage of burnout and ignoring it is how people sabotage themselves later through overcorrection or disengagement.

This is not the moment to push harder.Pushing harder assumes effort is the problem.Here the problem is capacity.

The correct response is **consolidation**: shifting to maintenance, stabilizing body composition, restoring training performance, normalizing appetite, and allowing psychological pressure to ease.

Progress is not lost during this phase.It is protected.

Recomposition works best in cycles. Knowing when to exit is what allows you to re-enter later with more capacity, better recovery, and fewer mental scars.

Chapter 19
How to Exit a Deficit Without Rebounding

Most rebound weight gain is not metabolic. It is behavioral.

People don't regain fat because their metabolism is "broken." They regain fat because they move from restraint to freedom overnight, assuming the work is finished and the rules no longer apply. The body responds predictably: appetite overshoots, structure collapses, and weight climbs faster than expected.

The solution is not fear.It is a controlled transition.

The Maintenance Ramp

Instead of jumping straight to unrestricted eating, exit the deficit gradually:

- Increase calories by **100–150 kcal**

- Hold for **7–10 days**

- Monitor:

    - Weekly average bodyweight

    - Waist measurement

    - Training performance

- Repeat until weight stabilizes and hunger normalizes

This ramp allows glycogen, hormones, and training output to recover without triggering compensatory overeating. Most lifters are surprised by how little food is required to feel dramatically better once the deficit truly ends.

What Weight Gain Is Normal?

Expect:

- **1–3 lb increase** from glycogen and water

- Fuller muscles

- Better pumps and training performance

This is not fat regain.It is fuel restoration.

Panicking at this stage—cutting calories again, adding cardio, tightening rules—is how people undo months of work. The scale is not signaling failure. It is signaling repletion.

The goal is not to stop weight from ever rising.The goal is to stop reacting emotionally when it does.

Chapter 20
Living at Maintenance Like an Adult

Maintenance is where many lifters feel lost—not because it's ineffective, but because it removes urgency.

There is no looming deadline. No aggressive deficit to chase. No dramatic weekly change to react to. The familiar feedback loop—scale drops, visible leanness, hunger as "proof of effort"—goes quiet.

That quiet is unsettling.

Without pressure, many lifters mistake calm for stagnation. Without rapid feedback, they assume something must be wrong. But nothing is wrong. That stillness is the point.

Maintenance strips away the illusion that progress only counts when it hurts. It forces you to train, eat, and recover without emotional urgency driving every decision. You're no longer reacting—you're practicing.

This phase teaches skills most people never develop:

- Holding structure without intensity

- Respecting signals instead of overriding them

- Trusting consistency over validation

Maintenance is not exciting, but it is honest. It shows you whether your routine fits your life—or only works under artificial pressure. It's where performance stabilizes, appetite normalizes, and the body learns that its current state is safe.

If maintenance feels boring, directionless, or quiet, that's not a flaw. That's the environment where progress becomes durable instead of fragile.

What Maintenance Actually Means

Maintenance is not:

- Perfect eating

- Daily tracking

- Avoiding enjoyment

Maintenance is:

- Stable bodyweight over time

- Consistent training

- Flexible nutrition within boundaries

Maintenance should feel lighter. Energy returns. Training feels reliable. Food choices stop carrying emotional weight. You're no longer negotiating hunger, fatigue, or guilt—you're functioning.

If maintenance feels stressful or rigid, the deficit never truly ended. Calories may be higher on paper, but mentally or behaviorally, you're still dieting.

Until that load is released, progress cannot be stabilized—only postponed.

How to Eat at Maintenance

Simple rules outperform complex ones:

- Keep protein consistent

- Eat carbohydrates to support training

- Let fats fluctuate naturally

- Track occasionally, not obsessively

Daily precision is fragile. Behavioral consistency is durable. When habits are steady, small imperfections don't matter because the pattern holds.

Progress comes from what you repeat, not what you perfect.

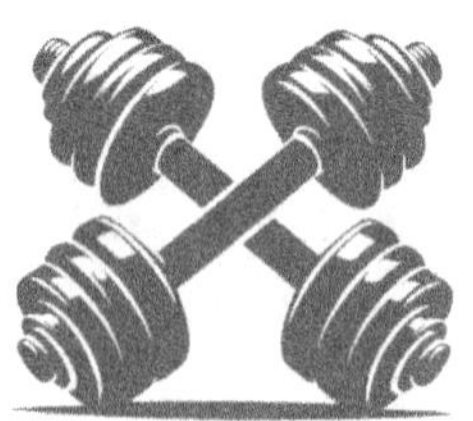

Chapter 21
Bulking

Should You Ever Bulk Again?

For many lifters, traditional bulking is unnecessary—and in some cases, counterproductive. The classic cycle of aggressive surplus followed by an equally aggressive cut is often treated as a rite of passage, but it is not a requirement for long-term progress.

Bulking assumes that faster weight gain equals faster muscle gain. In practice, that assumption rarely holds outside of very specific conditions.

If you are not already lean, if your recovery capacity is limited, or if training consistency is the primary constraint in your progress, pushing calories higher often creates more friction than momentum. Fat gain accelerates, conditioning erodes, and the psychological cost of "getting sloppy" begins to outweigh any marginal benefit in muscle accrual.

Muscle can still be built at or near maintenance. The process is slower, but it is cleaner. Strength can increase, tissue can be added, and performance can improve without the emotional whiplash that aggressive bulks tend to create.

Progress does not require excess. It requires consistency.

When a Bulk Makes Sense

A caloric surplus is not inherently wrong—it is simply situational. Bulking tends to work best when several conditions are already in place.

If you are already lean, recovery is robust, training performance is progressing, and you are willing to accept some degree of fat gain, a surplus can accelerate muscle growth. In that context, additional calories are more likely to be partitioned toward lean tissue rather than stored as fat.

Even then, "bulk" does not need to mean reckless. Surpluses that are small and controlled are far more productive than those driven by impatience.

When these conditions are not met, pushing food higher usually creates more problems than progress. Strength stalls under fatigue, body composition worsens, and the eventual cut becomes longer and more punishing than the bulk was productive.

The Recomposition Cycle Alternative

For many lifters, a cyclical recomposition model produces better long-term results with fewer setbacks. This approach prioritizes long periods at or near maintenance, punctuated by short, controlled fat-loss phases and occasional, modest surpluses when conditions truly support them.

The benefits are not dramatic, but they are durable.

Maintenance phases preserve muscle and performance. Short deficits minimize metabolic slowdown and reduce the risk of muscle loss. Small surpluses allow for incremental growth without significant fat regain. Over time, body composition improves not through extremes, but through accumulation.

This approach also reduces psychological burnout. There is no prolonged period of discomfort, no need to "undo" months of excess, and no identity shift between bulk and cut. Training remains the constant.

It is not flashy.It does not photograph well on social media.But it works.

How to Decide What Phase You're In

Most lifters don't stall because they chose the wrong strategy. They stall because they change strategies too often, or for the wrong reasons. Decision-making should be slow, evidence-based, and boring.

Before adjusting anything, answer one question honestly:

What is actually happening—not what you're afraid is happening?

That answer determines the phase.

Stay at Maintenance If...

Maintenance is not a holding pattern. It is an active phase, and for many lifters, it is where the majority of progress should occur.

Remain at maintenance if:

- Strength is stable or increasing

- Waist measurements are slowly decreasing or holding

- Recovery feels manageable

- Motivation and training consistency are high

This is not stagnation. This is recomposition working quietly. Changing phases here often interrupts progress that hasn't finished unfolding.

If nothing is breaking, do not try to fix it.

Enter a Short Deficit If...

Deficits are tools, not lifestyles. They exist to correct drift—not to chase leanness endlessly.

A short, controlled deficit makes sense when:

- Waist measurements are trending upward

- Conditioning is clearly declining

- Strength is stable enough to protect

- You can commit to a defined endpoint

The goal is correction, not punishment. Exit the deficit as soon as the signal improves. Staying longer rarely improves outcomes and often degrades performance.

Fat loss should feel intentional—not desperate.

Consider a Small Surplus If...

Surpluses are earned, not default.

A small surplus may be appropriate when:

- You are already lean

- Training performance is progressing

- Recovery is consistently strong

- Appetite, sleep, and stress are well controlled

Even then, the surplus should be modest and temporary. If fat gain outpaces performance gains, the experiment has failed—end it.

Growth that creates future cleanup work is rarely efficient.

The Governing Rule

Only one variable changes at a time.Only one phase is active at a time.Only objective signals—not emotion—trigger transitions.

Recomposition is not about finding the perfect phase. It's about staying in the *right* phase long enough for the body to respond.

Patience is not passive here.It is the strategy.

Chapter 22
Real Life

No plan survives real life perfectly.

This is not a personal failing—it is a structural reality. Training plans assume predictable schedules. Nutrition targets assume consistent access, sleep, and stress. Real life ignores all of that.

Travel disrupts routines.Work stress compresses recovery.Social events alter food choices.Illness, injury, and fatigue appear without warning.

The mistake most lifters make is interpreting these disruptions as emergencies.

They respond with urgency—cutting calories aggressively, adding extra sessions, or tightening rules beyond sustainability. This reaction is rarely rational. It is emotional, driven by the fear that progress is fragile and must be defended at all costs.

That belief is what actually causes regression.

Progress is not preserved through rigidity.It is preserved through *self-correction*.

A well-built physique is resilient. A few unstructured days do not erase months of consistent training and eating. Temporary weight fluctuations, missed sessions, or imperfect meals are not threats—they are noise. Treating them as crises teaches the body and mind that stability is conditional and easily lost.

Calm response is what keeps progress intact.

Self-correction means returning to baseline without drama. You don't compensate. You don't punish. You don't escalate. You simply resume the behaviors that created progress in the first place.

This approach requires trust—trust that your process works, trust that your body responds predictably over time, and trust that restraint is most effective when it is selective, not constant.

The ability to self-correct without panic is the clearest sign that recomposition has succeeded. It means progress no longer depends on perfect weeks or flawless execution. It depends on your capacity to re-center when life inevitably pulls you off course.

That capacity—not discipline, not intensity—is what makes results last.

Applied Example: A "Bad" Week That Isn't

Imagine a week where several things go wrong at once.

You travel for work. Training sessions are shortened or skipped. Meals are eaten out, portions are larger, sodium is higher, and tracking is inconsistent. Sleep is poor. By the end of the week, bodyweight is up three pounds, and you feel flat, bloated, and frustrated.

The common response is immediate correction:

- Slash calories

- Add extra cardio

- Push training volume to "make up for it"

This response feels responsible, but it is driven by fear, not evidence.

The correct response is simpler.

You return home. You resume normal training. You eat your usual meals. You do nothing aggressive for several days.

Within a week, water weight drops. Glycogen normalizes. Appetite stabilizes. Performance returns. The "gain" resolves without intervention because it was never fat to begin with—it was disruption.

Nothing was fixed because nothing was broken.

This is what self-correction looks like in practice. Not control, not punishment, not urgency—just a calm return to baseline. When this becomes your default response, setbacks stop feeling dangerous, and progress stops feeling fragile.

Consistency beats intensity every time.

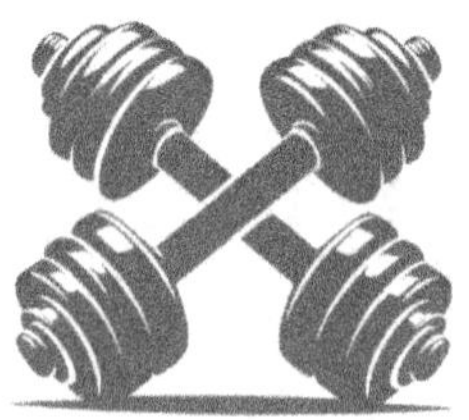

Chapter 23
The Real Goal of Recomposition

Recomposition is not about being lean forever.

Chasing permanent leanness turns physique improvement into a defensive exercise—one that requires constant vigilance, escalating control, and fear of deviation. That mindset doesn't create confidence. It creates fragility.

Recomposition is about changing your relationship with progress.

Instead of treating progress as something that must always move forward—or else be lost—you learn how to hold it. How to pause without panic. How to resume without starting over. The body becomes something you manage skillfully, not something you constantly pressure into compliance.

The real success is not visual.It is behavioral.

It shows up as:

- **Not restarting every year**, because you no longer rely on extremes that collapse under real life

- **Not fearing food**, because eating is no longer tied to guilt, urgency, or loss of control

- **Not chasing extremes**, because you understand that intensity is a tool, not a requirement

- **Trusting your ability to adjust calmly** because you know small corrections work when applied consistently

When these shifts occur, progress stops feeling fragile. Missed sessions, imperfect weeks, or changes in routine no longer trigger escalation. You respond instead of react. You correct instead of punish.

At that point, physique improvement becomes a side effect—not a struggle.

Leanness comes and goes. Muscle accumulates slowly. Body composition shifts over time. None of it requires constant force once the underlying skills are in place.

That is what this process was for.

Not a body that demands permanent discipline,but one that remains stable because you know how to live inside it.

Epilogue
What Changes When This Finally Works

If you've read this far, you already know the truth most people avoid: the problem was never information.It was escalation.

More rules.More urgency.More punishment when progress slowed.

I want to step outside the science for a moment.

Ten years ago I weighed 350 pounds. Today I weigh around 245 — but the number is almost beside the point. What I care about is whether my body is lean and strong. It is. Could it be leaner? Yes. Am I still working on that? Yes. My body fat currently sits around 23%. The average American male my age carries around 29%. I am working toward the teens and I know I will get there. But like the tortoise, progress is slow — and the closer you get, the slower it becomes. That is not the moment to get discouraged. That is the moment to turn around and look at how far you have come.

Did it take ten years? Not really. I didn't start in earnest until about seven years ago. Age plays a role — metabolism slows, macros have to be tighter, the margins get narrower. But it can be done. I am living proof of that, and I am considerably healthier at 65 than I was at 55.

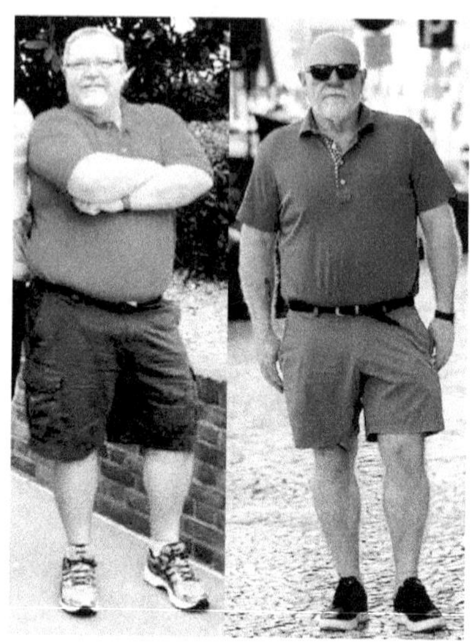

I also have chronic insomnia. On nights when I sleep three hours, I don't push hard at the gym. I can't. The body doesn't negotiate with circumstances — it simply responds to them. Training stress, work stress, the stress of a difficult week — the body processes all of it through the same systems. The only way through is rest, adequate nutrition, and sleep when sleep will come. Many people, myself included, benefit from therapy. Decompression is not weakness. It is part of the process.

This book has not given you a faster way to change your body. It has given you a *quieter* one. One that respects physiology, acknowledges psychology, and stops mistaking suffering for effectiveness.

When recomposition finally works, something subtle but important happens. Food loses its power to provoke anxiety or excitement. Training stops feeling like a referendum on your worth. Progress becomes something you manage, not something you chase.

You stop asking, *"What can I add?"* You start asking, *"What can I sustain?"*

That shift changes everything.

You no longer need constant novelty or pressure to stay engaged. You don't need extreme deficits to feel legitimate. You don't need to restart every time life interrupts your plan. You know how to slow down, how to stabilize, and how to reapply effort only when it makes sense.

Most importantly, you trust yourself again.

That trust is what prevents rebound—not a macro target, not a rule set, not discipline theater. It's the confidence that you can respond instead of react. Adjust instead of overcorrect. Pause instead of panic.

This is why the end of recomposition is intentionally anticlimactic. There is no dramatic finish line. No final reveal. Just a body that feels easier to maintain and a process that no longer requires heroics.

That's not a lack of payoff. That *is* the payoff.

From here, progress becomes optional instead of urgent. You can pursue more muscle, more leanness, or simply more capacity for life—without fear that everything will unravel if you ease off.

That's the real result most people never reach.

Not a physique that demands constant defense. But one that stays because you know how to live inside it.

And once you understand that, you don't need another plan.

You're done starting over.

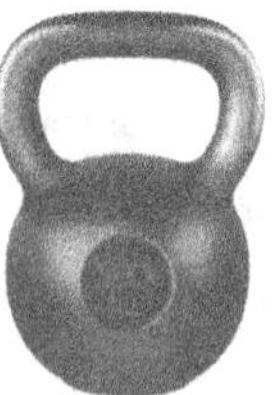

Appendices

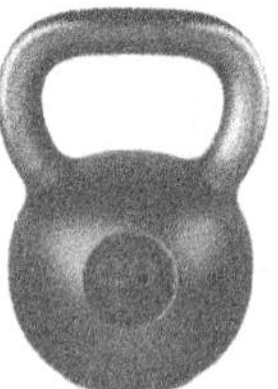

Appendix 1
FAQs

1. Is the goal of this approach simply to lose weight?

No. The goal is to improve body composition, not just reduce body weight. Many diets succeed in making people lighter but fail to make them healthier or stronger. The Durable Physique approach prioritizes fat loss while preserving muscle, because muscle is what gives the body its metabolic stability and physical capability.

2. Why do most weight-loss programs fail?

Most programs rely on large calorie deficits and extreme behavioral changes. These approaches can produce rapid early results but are difficult to maintain. Eventually hunger, fatigue, and lifestyle friction overwhelm the plan. A durable approach favors moderate deficits and repeatable habits that can be sustained for months and years.

3. Why is muscle preservation so important during fat loss?

When calories drop, the body will lose both fat and muscle unless it receives signals to preserve lean tissue. Muscle is critical for strength, metabolic health, and long-term weight maintenance. Losing significant muscle during dieting often results in a smaller but weaker body that struggles to maintain its new weight.

4. Can I improve my body composition without lifting weights?

It is possible to lose fat without resistance training, but it is much harder to maintain muscle mass without it. Resistance training provides the signal that tells the body to preserve lean tissue. Even modest strength training dramatically improves the quality of weight loss.

5. How much protein do I actually need?

Most people benefit from roughly 0.6–0.8 grams of protein per pound of body weight, or about 0.7–1.0 grams per pound of lean body mass. This range supports muscle maintenance during caloric deficits and improves recovery from training.

6. Do I need to track calories or macros?

Strict tracking is not mandatory, but it is often helpful. Many people underestimate their intake without realizing it. Tracking—at least temporarily—can provide the awareness necessary to understand energy balance and portion sizes.

7. What is a reasonable calorie deficit?

For most people, a daily deficit of 300–500 calories is sufficient to promote steady fat loss without significantly impairing energy levels, training performance, or recovery.

8. Should I use bulk-and-cut cycles to build muscle?

Traditional bulk-and-cut cycles often encourage unnecessary fat gain followed by aggressive dieting. Many individuals can gradually improve body composition through consistent resistance training, adequate protein, and moderate calorie control, avoiding large swings in body weight.

9. How much cardio should I do?

Cardio is valuable for cardiovascular health, endurance, and overall activity levels. However, nutrition and resistance training play a much larger role in shaping body composition. Cardio should support health, not function as punishment for eating.

10. Do I need a personal trainer?

No. You do not need a personal trainer to build a durable physique. The principles that drive long-term progress—consistent resistance training, adequate protein, moderate calorie control, and recovery—can be followed independently.

That said, life is often easier with one. A good trainer can teach proper technique, structure effective workouts, and provide accountability. The right coach can shorten the learning curve and help you avoid common mistakes, but long-term success ultimately depends on the habits you maintain yourself.

11. How often should I train?

Most people make excellent progress training three to four days per week. Consistency and recoverable workload matter more than extreme training frequency.

12. What is recoverable training volume?

Recoverable training volume refers to the amount of training stress your body can adapt to and recover from consistently. Training beyond recovery capacity often leads to fatigue, stalled progress, and injury. Sustainable progress comes from workloads you can repeat week after week.

13. How fast should fat loss occur?

A sustainable rate of fat loss for most people is roughly 0.5–1 percent of body weight per week. Faster weight loss usually increases the risk of muscle loss and poor adherence.

14. Why does the scale sometimes stop moving?

Fat loss is rarely linear. Water retention, glycogen changes, stress, and hormonal fluctuations can temporarily mask fat loss. Plateaus are common and do not necessarily indicate that progress has stopped.

15. How do I break through a plateau?

Plateaus typically resolve by making small adjustments, such as modestly reducing calorie intake, increasing daily activity, or progressing training stimulus. Large, drastic changes are rarely necessary.

16. Can beginners gain muscle while losing fat?

Yes. Individuals who are new to resistance training often experience a period where muscle gain and fat loss occur simultaneously, especially when protein intake and training stimulus increase.

17. Do I need supplements to succeed?

Supplements are optional. The fundamentals—nutrition, resistance training, sleep, and consistency—produce the vast majority of results. Supplements may offer minor support, but they cannot replace these fundamentals.

18. What role does sleep play in body composition?

Sleep affects hunger regulation, training performance, recovery, and metabolic health. Chronic sleep deprivation increases appetite and reduces training quality. Consistently sleeping seven to nine hours per night improves adherence and long-term outcomes.

19. Will slow fat loss leave me with loose skin?

Loose skin is influenced by age, genetics, the duration of obesity, and the amount of weight lost. Slower fat loss and resistance training may improve skin appearance, but some individuals will still experience loose skin after large weight reductions.

20. What body fat percentage should I aim for?

Healthy and sustainable ranges vary, but many men feel and perform well around 12–18 percent body fat, and many women around 20–28 percent. The goal is not extreme leanness but a body that is strong, functional, and maintainable.

21. What happens once I reach my goal?

The habits that built the Durable Physique are the same habits that maintain it. Rather than abandoning structure, gradually transition toward maintenance calories while continuing resistance training and adequate protein intake.

22. How long does it take to build a durable physique?

Meaningful body recomposition usually occurs over years, not weeks. The Durable Physique is the product of steady habits repeated over long periods of time.

23. What defines a durable physique?

A durable physique is not defined by temporary aesthetics but by long-term capability. It is a body that remains strong, metabolically healthy, and functional across decades because it was built through sustainable practices rather than extreme interventions.

Appendix 2
Glossary

Adherence — Your ability to follow the plan consistently over time; the practical limiter of most diets and training programs.

Adaptation — The body's response to training stress (stronger, more skilled, more muscular) that only happens when recovery resources are available.

Adaptation resistance — When training stimulus is present but calories/recovery are too low for the body to respond; progress stalls despite effort.

Aggressive deficit — A large calorie shortfall (often from severe restriction) that speeds scale loss but increases fatigue, hunger, and muscle-loss risk.

Allostatic load — The total accumulated stress load (training + work + life + sleep loss) that draws from the same recovery "budget."

Amino acids — The building blocks of protein used to repair and maintain lean tissue.

Anabolic window — The idea you must eat protein/carbs within a short time post-workout or "miss gains"; described here as largely outdated.

Beginner luck — Early improvements in strength/physique from new training; recomposition can happen beyond this, but the margin for error narrows.

Bioavailability — How efficiently a protein source is digested and used; animal proteins are described as generally more bioavailable.

Body recomposition — Simultaneous fat loss and muscle maintenance (or slow gain), emphasizing tissue quality over rapid scale changes.

Bulk — A phase of eating more to gain muscle while accepting fat gain; portrayed as often drifting into overeating for non-elite lifters.

Bulk/cut trap — The repeated cycle of bulking and cutting that often leads natural lifters to lose muscle, regain fat, and end up smaller and frustrated.

Calorie deficit — Eating fewer calories than you expend; required for fat loss, but the size and "cost" of the deficit matters.

Calorie tolerance — How many calories you can eat while still progressing or maintaining; tends to decline when muscle is lost.

Carb cycling (training days vs rest days) — Modestly higher calories/carbs on training days and slightly lower on rest days to match demand, not "confuse" the body.

Carbohydrates (carbs) — Primary training fuel for lifters because they replenish glycogen and support performance and recovery.

Catabolic environment — A deficit state where muscle breakdown rises and muscle building/maintenance is harder to stimulate.

Chronic kidney disease (CKD) — The population where high protein may be harmful; the text distinguishes this from healthy lifters.

Conditioning — Cardio/fitness work; helpful when it supports lifting and adherence, harmful when it competes with recovery.

Consistency — Repeating the essentials long enough for trends to appear; framed as the decisive factor over intensity or novelty.

Cut — A fat-loss phase of eating less; commonly associated with some muscle loss when deficits are too aggressive.

Decimals (scale false precision) — The misleading feeling that daily 0.2–0.4 lb changes are meaningful; daily weight is noisy.

Deficit size — How large the calorie shortfall is; small-to-moderate deficits are positioned as best for recomposition outcomes.

Diet fatigue — The accumulated mental/physical strain of prolonged restriction (hunger, irritability, burnout signals).

Dietary fat — Essential for hormones, vitamin absorption, satiety; treated as a "baseline to respect" and easy to overconsume.

Diminishing returns (protein) — Past a useful intake level, extra protein doesn't keep improving outcomes and may crowd out carbs/fats.

Energy balance — The rule that fat loss requires a deficit and gain requires surplus; recomposition doesn't "break" this.

Enhanced athletes — Drug-assisted lifters with increased recovery capacity; the book is positioned as *not* for them.

Execution quality — Controlled reps and technique that ensure the target muscle carries the load (a key part of mechanical tension).

Failure (training to failure) — Completing reps until you can't do another; has a place but can be too fatiguing if used constantly in a deficit.

Fat regain — Post-diet rebound driven mostly by behavior and appetite overshoot; easier after muscle loss and hard dieting.

Framework problem — The idea that most lifters fail not from laziness but because the overall system doesn't align training, nutrition, and recovery.

Fuel restoration — The expected 1–3 lb weight gain after a deficit from glycogen/water returning; not the same as fat regain.

Ghrelin — "Hunger hormone" that rises with energy shortage and poor sleep, increasing appetite and food focus.

Glycogen — Stored carbohydrate in muscle used heavily during lifting; low glycogen makes sets feel heavier and volume tolerance drop.

HIIT (high-intensity interval training) — Higher fatigue cardio; cautioned as often too recovery-costly when paired with hard lifting and a deficit.

Hormonal regulation — The recovery/appetite/stress hormone environment (testosterone, cortisol, leptin/ghrelin) influenced strongly by sleep and deficits.

Intensity (training) — How hard sets are relative to max effort; paired with proximity to failure to create tension without excessive fatigue.

Junk volume — Extra sets/work that create fatigue without meaningful stimulus; especially harmful when recovery is limited.

Lean mass — Muscle and other non-fat tissue; preserving it is framed as the foundation of a durable physique.

Leptin — Satiety/energy sufficiency signal produced by fat cells; decreases during dieting and with poor sleep, making hunger harder to manage.

LISS (low-intensity steady-state) — Low-fatigue cardio (walking, cycling) described as most compatible with recomposition.

Maintenance — A phase of stable intake and bodyweight; framed as strategic consolidation, not quitting.

Maintenance ramp — Gradual post-diet calorie increases (100–150 kcal steps, 7–10 days each) to stabilize appetite and weight without rebound.

Mechanical tension — The primary driver of muscle retention/growth: challenging loads + controlled execution + close-enough effort.

Metabolic adaptation — Normal reductions in energy expenditure and activity during dieting; not "metabolic damage," but a predictable response.

Metabolic circuits / "fat-burning" training — High-rep, sweaty conditioning-style workouts that feel hard but may dilute tension and increase recovery cost.

Modest deficit — Smaller calorie shortfall that keeps performance and recovery intact; repeatedly positioned as superior for recomposition.

Nutrient partitioning — How the body allocates resources; recomposition improves partitioning so more goes to muscle repair and less to fat.

Non-exercise activity (NEAT) — Unconscious daily movement that often decreases during dieting, reducing total expenditure.

Natural lifter — Drug-free lifter; the primary audience the text is written for.

Overcorrection — Making big reactive changes (slashing calories, adding cardio) based on short-term noise; a major recomposition killer.

Performance (as a metric) — Loads, reps, sets, effort; the clearest proxy for muscle retention during fat loss.

Perceived plateau — A temporary stall caused by water, stress, cycle fluctuations, or tracking noise; solved by time, not panic.

Plateau (true) — No movement in weekly average weight, measurements, and visuals for ~4+ weeks with consistent adherence; requires a small adjustment.

Protein (non-negotiable) — The top nutritional priority for recomposition; supports muscle repair/retention and improves satiety.

Protein distribution — Spreading protein across the day (3–5 meals, ~25–40 g/meal) to support muscle protein synthesis and satiety.

Protein targets (evidence-based ranges) — ~0.6–0.8 g/lb bodyweight for most, or ~0.7–1.0 g/lb lean body mass; higher end for lean/aggressive/hard-training.

Proximity to failure / RIR — How close a set is to max reps; 1–3 reps in reserve is described as the sweet spot for recomposition.

Recovery capacity — The amount of training stress you can absorb and adapt to; reduced in a deficit and under high life stress.

Reps in reserve (RIR) — A way to gauge effort: how many reps you could still do at the end of a set.

Resistance training — The core "signal" that muscle is still required; without it, fat loss tends to include muscle loss.

Resting energy expenditure — Calories burned at rest; often declines with muscle loss and dieting, making future fat loss harder.

Scale obsession — Treating daily weigh-ins as verdicts; leads to emotional decisions and worse outcomes.

Scale trend (weekly averages) — A better use of the scale: look at averages and 3–4 week trends rather than daily fluctuations.

Self-correction — Returning to baseline habits calmly after disruptions (travel, missed sessions) without punishment or escalation.

Signal (training signal) — The body's reason to keep muscle: repeated mechanical tension and stable performance.

Sustainability — The ability to maintain the approach without life being consumed by dieting; positioned as a core priority.

Tissue quality — The meaningful outcome (more muscle, less fat) versus mere weight change.

Training demand alignment — Matching calorie/carbohydrate intake to how hard you're training; mismatches stall progress.

Training frequency — How often you train a muscle; twice per week is positioned as generally better than once.

Training volume — Total hard sets; recommended working range given as ~8–15 hard sets per muscle group per week (adjusted by recovery).

True progress signals (the "big three") — Waist/measurements, performance, and weight trend (in that order of usefulness, per the text).

Volume creep — The gradual, often unconscious increase in training volume when gains slow; especially destructive in a deficit.

Waist measurement — A key recomposition indicator; shrinking waist with stable bodyweight signals fat loss with muscle retention.

Appendix 3
Supplements: Necessary, Optional, and Unnecessary

Supplements are not a foundation. They are, at best, small modifiers layered on top of consistent training, adequate nutrition, and sufficient recovery. When those fundamentals are missing, supplements do nothing. When they are in place, a few select compounds can provide modest but reliable benefits.

Most lifters dramatically overestimate what supplements can do—and underestimate how little they need.

Supplements Worth Using

These are the few supplements with consistent evidence, meaningful upside, and minimal downside when used correctly.

Protein Powder

Protein powder is not magic—it is convenience. Its only function is to help meet daily protein targets reliably and efficiently.

It is useful if:

- Whole-food protein intake is inconsistent

- Appetite is low

- Time or logistics are limiting

It is unnecessary if protein needs are already met through food. The benefit comes from protein itself, not the delivery system.

Creatine Monohydrate

Creatine is one of the most studied and effective performance supplements available.

Benefits include:

- Improved strength and power output

- Increased training volume capacity

- Small increases in lean mass over time

Dose is simple: 3–5 grams daily. Timing is irrelevant. Cycling is unnecessary. Creatine works slowly, quietly, and reliably—which is exactly what you want.

Caffeine (Strategic Use)

Caffeine improves alertness, perceived effort, and short-term performance. Used correctly, it can enhance training quality.

Used poorly, it disrupts sleep, increases anxiety, and masks fatigue.

Best practices:

- Use sparingly, not daily

- Avoid late-day intake

- Do not rely on it to compensate for poor recovery

Caffeine is a tool, not a crutch.

Vitamin D (Context-Dependent)

Vitamin D may be beneficial if levels are low, which is common in individuals with limited sun exposure.

This is not a blanket recommendation. Blood work—not guesswork—should guide supplementation when possible.

More is not better. Correct deficiency, then reassess.

Supplements That Are Optional (Low Impact, Situational)

These supplements may offer small benefits in specific contexts, but they do not meaningfully change outcomes.

Omega-3 Fatty Acids

May support general health and inflammation management, especially if dietary intake of fatty fish is low. Effects on body composition and performance are modest at best.

Helpful for health. Not transformative for recomposition.

Electrolytes

Useful during:

- Heavy sweating

- High-volume training

- Hot environments

- Low-carbohydrate phases

Unnecessary for most lifters eating a normal diet and training indoors.

Magnesium

May support sleep quality or muscle relaxation in individuals who are deficient. Effects vary widely.

If sleep is poor, address sleep hygiene before adding supplements.

Supplements You Can Ignore

These supplements are aggressively marketed, weakly supported, or entirely unnecessary.

Fat Burners

Fat burners do not burn fat. At best, they are caffeine blends with added stimulants. At worst, they increase stress, disrupt sleep, and worsen adherence.

Fat loss comes from energy balance, not capsules.

Testosterone Boosters

Over-the-counter testosterone boosters do not meaningfully increase testosterone in healthy men. If testosterone is clinically low, supplements will not fix it.

Lifestyle factors—sleep, stress, nutrition—matter more than any pill.

BCAAs and EAAs (In Most Cases)

If total protein intake is adequate, amino acid supplements provide no additional benefit. They are redundant.

Drink protein or eat food instead.

Detoxes, Cleanses, and Hormone "Resets"

These are marketing constructs, not physiological necessities. The liver and kidneys already perform detoxification effectively.

If a product promises to "reset" your hormones, it is selling a story—not a mechanism.

The Guiding Principle

Supplements should solve a specific problem. If you cannot clearly articulate the problem they are addressing, you do not need them.

Most progress comes from:

- Training consistency

- Sufficient protein

- Adequate calories

- Quality sleep

Everything else is marginal.

Appendix 4
Muscle Groups

Major Muscle Groups: Common and Medical Names

Chest

- **Common name:** Chest

- **Medical name:** *Pectoralis major*

- **Primary function:** Horizontal adduction of the shoulder, pushing movements

Upper Back

- **Common name:** Lats

- **Medical name:** *Latissimus dorsi*

- **Primary function:** Shoulder extension, adduction, pulling movements

- **Common name:** Upper back

- **Medical names:** *Trapezius* (upper, middle, lower fibers), *Rhomboid major/minor*

- **Primary function:** Scapular elevation, retraction, depression, stability

Shoulders

- **Common name:** Delts / Shoulders

- **Medical name:** *Deltoid* (anterior, lateral, posterior heads)

- **Primary function:** Shoulder flexion, abduction, extension, rotation

Arms (Upper)

Biceps

- **Common name:** Biceps

- **Medical name:** *Biceps brachii*

- **Primary function:** Elbow flexion, forearm supination

Triceps

- **Common name:** Triceps

- **Medical name:** *Triceps brachii*

- **Primary function:** Elbow extension

Forearms

- **Common name:** Forearms

- **Medical names:** *Flexor* and *extensor muscle groups of the forearm*

- **Primary function:** Wrist and finger flexion/extension, grip strength

Core / Trunk

Abdominals

- **Common name:** Abs

- **Medical names:** *Rectus abdominis, External obliques, Internal obliques, Transversus abdominis*

- **Primary function:** Trunk flexion, rotation, bracing, spinal stability

Lower Back
- **Common name:** Lower back

- **Medical name:** *Erector spinae*

- **Primary function:** Spinal extension, posture, load tolerance

Hips & Glutes
- **Common name:** Glutes

- **Medical names:** *Gluteus maximus, Gluteus medius, Gluteus minimus*

- **Primary function:** Hip extension, abduction, pelvic stability

Thighs (Upper Leg)
Quads
- **Common name:** Quads

- **Medical name:** *Quadriceps femoris*

  - (Rectus femoris, Vastus lateralis, Vastus medialis, Vastus intermedius)

- **Primary function:** Knee extension

Hamstrings
- **Common name:** Hamstrings

- **Medical names:** *Biceps femoris, Semitendinosus, Semimembranosus*

- **Primary function:** Knee flexion, hip extension

Adductors
- **Common name:** Inner thighs

- **Medical names:** *Adductor longus, brevis, magnus, Gracilis*

- **Primary function:** Hip adduction, pelvic control

Lower Legs

Calves

- **Common name:** Calves

- **Medical names:** *Gastrocnemius, Soleus*

- **Primary function:** Ankle plantarflexion, gait and jumping mechanics

Shins

- **Common name:** Shins

- **Medical name:** *Tibialis anterior*

- **Primary function:** Ankle dorsiflexion, foot clearance during walking/running

While anatomy textbooks divide the body into dozens of muscles, training adapts tissue based on **function and loading**, not memorization. For recomposition purposes, these major groups represent the **primary drivers of strength, physique change, and metabolic demand.**

You do not need to know every muscle. You need to train the important ones well.

This focus is on body recomposition for natural lifters—fat loss that preserves muscle, strength, and performance while respecting recovery and real life. Rather than chasing rapid weight loss or extreme phases, my work prioritizes durability: progress that survives stress, imperfect weeks, and the transition out of dieting.

My approach is grounded in exercise physiology, nutrition science, and long-term coaching principles, but filtered through a practical lens. If a method produces results that can't be maintained—or requires repeated cycles of breakdown and repair—it isn't durable, and it isn't success.

This book is written for people who train seriously and want a physique that holds together over time. Not optimized for short-term transformation photos, but built to last.

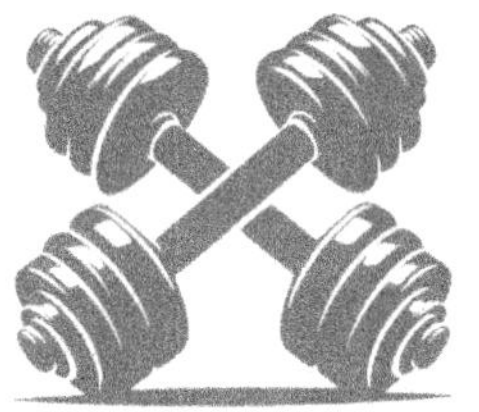

Appendix 5
References

Resistance Training, Volume, and Hypertrophy

- Dankel, S. J., et al. Mechanical tension and muscle hypertrophy: A review. Sports Medicine, 2017.

- Morton, R. W., et al. Training volume and muscle hypertrophy: A systematic review and meta-analysis. British Journal of Sports Medicine, 2019.

- Phillips, S. M. Resistance exercise and muscle protein synthesis. Journal of Applied Physiology, 2009.

- Schoenfeld, B. J. The mechanisms of muscle hypertrophy and their application to resistance training. Sports Medicine, 2010.

- Schoenfeld, B. J., et al. Resistance training volume enhances muscle hypertrophy but not strength in trained men. Journal of Strength and Conditioning Research, 2019.

Dieting, Energy Balance, and Metabolic Adaptation

- Byrne, N. M., et al. Metabolic adaptation following weight loss. The American Journal of Clinical Nutrition, 2018.

- Dulloo, A. G., et al. Adaptive thermogenesis in human body weight regulation. Obesity Reviews, 2015.

- Forbes, G. B. Lean body mass–fat interrelationships in humans. Nutrition Reviews, 1987.

- Garthe, I., et al. Effect of two different weight-loss rates on body composition and strength. International Journal of Sport Nutrition and Exercise Metabolism, 2011.

- Hall, K. D., et al. Energy balance and its components: Implications for body weight regulation. The American Journal of Clinical Nutrition, 2012.

- Heymsfield, S. B., et al. Energy balance: Myths and realities. The American Journal of Clinical Nutrition, 2014.

- Müller, M. J., et al. Metabolic adaptation to caloric restriction and consequences for weight loss maintenance. Obesity Reviews, 2015.

- Rosenbaum, M., Leibel, R. L. Adaptive thermogenesis in humans. International Journal of Obesity, 2010.

- Trexler, E. T., et al. Metabolic adaptation to weight loss: Implications for the athlete. Journal of the International Society of Sports Nutrition, 2014.

Protein Intake, Macronutrients, and Muscle Retention

- Antonio, J., et al. Common questions and misconceptions about protein supplementation. Journal of the International Society of Sports Nutrition, 2018.

- Helms, E. R., et al. Evidence-based recommendations for natural bodybuilding contest preparation. Journal of Sports Medicine, 2014.

- Morton, R. W., et al. Protein supplementation to enhance muscle hypertrophy. British Journal of Sports Medicine, 2018.

- Pasiakos, S. M., et al. Higher-protein diets preserve lean mass during weight loss. The American Journal of Clinical Nutrition, 2013.

- Phillips, S. M., Van Loon, L. J. C. Dietary protein for athletes. Journal of Sports Sciences, 2011.

- Schoenfeld, B. J., Aragon, A. A. How much protein can the body use in a single meal? Journal of the International Society of Sports Nutrition, 2018.

Carbohydrates, Glycogen, and Performance

- Burke, L. M., et al. Carbohydrates for training and competition. Journal of Sports Sciences, 2011.

- Helms, E. R., et al. Carbohydrate intake during contest preparation. Journal of the International Society of Sports Nutrition, 2014.

- Impey, S. G., et al. Fueling the work required: A theoretical framework for carbohydrate periodization. Sports Medicine, 2018.

- Slater, G., Phillips, S. M. Nutrition guidelines for strength sports. Strength and Conditioning Journal, 2011.

Dietary Fat, Hormones, and Satiety

- Astrup, A., et al. Dietary fat and body weight. The American Journal of Clinical Nutrition, 2011.

- Hall, K. D., et al. Calorie density and fat overconsumption. The American Journal of Clinical Nutrition, 2012.

- Jensen, M. D., et al. Dietary fats and health. Journal of Clinical Endocrinology & Metabolism, 2014.

- Volek, J. S., et al. Dietary fat intake and hormonal responses. Journal of Applied Physiology, 1997.

Sleep, Stress, and Recovery

- Dattilo, M., et al. Sleep and muscle recovery: Endocrinological and molecular basis. Medical Hypotheses, 2011.

- Halson, S. L. Sleep in elite athletes. Sports Medicine, 2014.

- Kellmann, M. Preventing overtraining and monitoring stress/recovery. Scandinavian Journal of Medicine & Science in Sports, 2010.

- Leproult, R., Van Cauter, E. Effect of sleep restriction on testosterone levels. JAMA, 2011.

- McEwen, B. S. Protective and damaging effects of stress mediators. New England Journal of Medicine, 1998.

- McEwen, B. S., Stellar, E. Stress and the individual: Mechanisms leading to disease. Archives of Internal Medicine, 1993.

- Meeusen, R., et al. Prevention, diagnosis, and treatment of overtraining syndrome. European Journal of Sport Science, 2013.

- Nedeltcheva, A. V., et al. Sleep curtailment and energy intake. The American Journal of Clinical Nutrition, 2009.

- Spiegel, K., et al. Impact of sleep debt on metabolic and endocrine function. The Lancet, 1999.

- Spiegel, K., et al. Sleep curtailment, leptin, ghrelin, and hunger. Annals of Internal Medicine, 2004.

- Taheri, S., et al. Short sleep duration and leptin/ghrelin. PLoS Medicine, 2004.

Concurrent Training, Cardio, and Interference

- Fyfe, J. J., et al. Interference effect of endurance training. Sports Medicine, 2014.

- Hickson, R. C. Interference of strength development by endurance training. European Journal of Applied Physiology, 1980.

- Wilson, J. M., et al. Concurrent training meta-analysis. Journal of Strength and Conditioning Research, 2012.